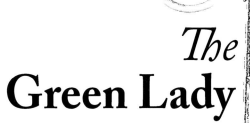

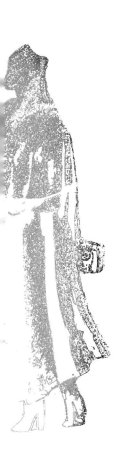

The
Green Lady

Memoirs of a Glasgow Midwife

Helena Joyce

2nd Edition

Ladysmith, Canada

The Green Lady: Memoirs of a Glasgow Midwife (2nd Edition)
A Turning Point Arts Book / August 2009

All rights reserved.

Copyright © 2008-2009, Helena Joyce, Richard Barnes

All rights are reserved under International and Pan-American Copyright Conventions. No part of this book may be reproduced in any form or by any electronic or mechanical means, including information storage and retrieval systems, without permission in writing from the author, except by a reviewer, who may quote brief passages in a review.

This is a work of creative nonfiction and depicts actual people, places and events. People's names have been fictionalized except where permission has been granted to use the actual names.

Library and Archives Canada Cataloguing in Publication

Joyce, Helena, 1939-

    The green lady : memoirs of a Glasgow midwife / Helena Joyce. -- 2nd ed.

ISBN 978-0-9812347-1-7

    1. Midwifery--Scotland--Glasgow--History--Fiction. 2. Childbirth at home--Scotland--Glasgow--History--Fiction. I. Title.

PS8619.O96G7 2009   C813'.6   C2009-903773-4

Anne Marzaroli has kindly granted permission to reproduce photographs from *Shades of Scotland 1956–1988* by Oscar Marzaroli and James Grassie, 1989.

Cover and chapter illustrations are copyright © 2008, Bradley A. Grigor, Turning Point Arts and its licensors. All rights reserved.

PRINTED IN CANADA

Dedication

To my daughters Morag and Sheila who encouraged me to write my memoirs way back in 2000, and without whom life for me would have been impossible.

Acknowledgements

I wish to thank:
- Anne Marzaroli for her kind permission to use her late husband Oscar Marzaroli's photography.
- The women I had the privilege to serve and to their families.
- My husband Richard, who encouraged me every step of the way.
- My late sister Evelyn, who did my early research in the Mitchell Library.
- My sisters Mary, Winnie and Nancy who have always been my confidants.
- Roy, Ian and Tony, my brothers-in-law, for being part of my research team.
- The Ladysmith Writer's Circle for their encouragement and editing services.
- Brad and Peggy Grigor for their inspiration and expertise in layout and design.
- My midwife friends for their encouragement.

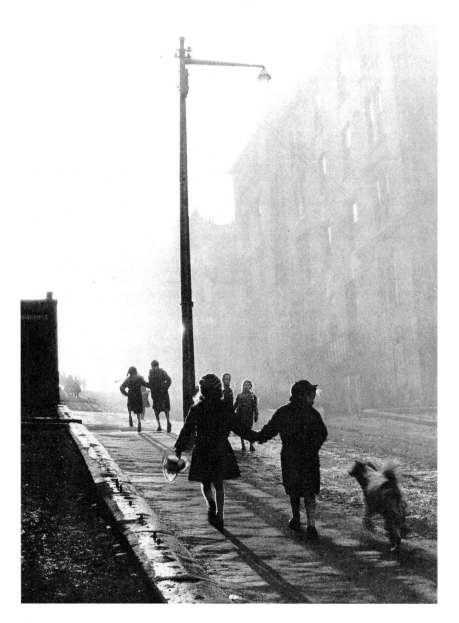

Foreword

In the 1960s, Helena Joyce worked as a Green Lady in Glasgow Scotland. You are about to read of those experiences through the eyes of her alter ego, Nell Dickson. Although there is no doubt that Helena was a superb nurse and midwife, the wonderful Glaswegian that I know and love is not the nurse, but the author, Helena Joyce.

We first met when I joined the Ladysmith Writers' Circle in 2005. Helena co-founded this small group several months earlier and set the mission statement to read, "To aid and abet those with a passion for writing." And Helena was as passionate about writing as she was about nursing. In 2006, with other members of the Writers' Circle, she helped pen, produce and market our first book, *Lines on the 49th Parallel*. When we picked up the first copy of that book, her childlike glee and enthusiasm were infectious. Helena was infectious.

The Green Lady stories came about from the urgings of her friends and family, who she had entertained for many years with tales of her rich and rewarding career as a midwife. Helena is quoted as saying, "To be divorced from my special memories as a young midwife in Glasgow by distance and time has made them more vivid and heartwarming, and has sparked my desire to write about them."

In 1997 she underwent hip surgery, which forced her to take time off from her busy career as a professor of maternity nursing. During her recovery, she started writing *The Green Lady* stories. Eight years later, when the Writers' Circle was formed, the stories were revived with an eye to publishing them.

In the spring of 2007, Helena visited Glasgow to listen to a speech given by her daughter, Sheila, also a midwife, at the National Midwifery Convention. While there, Helena made contact with her former colleagues and asked if she could present *The Green Lady* at the International Midwives Convention, scheduled to take place in Glasgow the following year. The answer was a resounding "yes!"

While in Glasgow, Helena had her first fainting spell and when she returned to Canada, she was given a pacemaker to correct an irregular heartbeat. But when the fainting spells persisted, it was discovered that she had a rare and deadly brain tumor known as Glioblastoma. The tumor was removed immediately, and a summer of intensive chemotherapy and radiation followed.

Instead of being deterred by this situation, Helena set herself three major goals. Sporting a tee shirt that read 'Glioblastoma has left the Building', she carried a notebook with these objectives written down, and repeated them over and over again, as a mantra, to everyone she met.

Her first goal was to be able to accompany her husband on a pre-planned South Seas Cruise encompassing Sydney and Melbourne Australia, Tasmania and New Zealand. Although weakened by her aggressive course of treatment, they did, indeed, embark on that cruise in February 2008.

Her second goal was to finish and publish *The Green Lady*. From September until April, Helena put this process into motion. She rounded up a team to help her do the final editing, design, layout and publishing of her book. She worked diligently on all the arrangements needed to make her dreams come true, working against a very challenging deadline that included having half the printing shipment sent to Scotland before the conference.

The task of producing a completed book, given a short and rigid deadline, is extremely challenging for anyone to accomplish, let alone someone with a serious illness. But Helena juggled the task around medical appointments, constant blood tests, researching anti-cancer strategies and hosting a barrage of concerned visitors from around the world. The book was published just in time, and arrived in Glasgow that April, only days before the conference.

That brings us to her third goal, which was to present *The Green Lady* in Glasgow at the aforementioned International Midwives Convention. Her crowning glory was when she stepped onto that stage in April 2008 to tell her beloved stories to modern day midwives, nurses and professors. She was so well received that Helena said the books literally 'flew off the table'. Her book continues to sell in Scotland and is carried, among other places, in the Glasgow museum, Mitchell Library and three midwifery schools.

To have been able to rally up the strength and determination to achieve these monumental tasks, while fighting for her very life, is a testament to

Helena's unwavering determination and strength of character. She was known to say that once she got her "Scottish up", there was no stopping her!

Her victorious return home inspired her to begin to pen a sequel, and in the months that followed, she put together many more Green Lady stories. In September 2008, Helena went for an MRI and was declared cancer free. With renewed vitality, she continued her writing and we, her publishing team, decided that it was time to start promoting *The Green Lady* in Canada, even though she had almost sold out of her original print run. In November, she did a reading and book launch at the Ladysmith library, the home of the Writers' Circle.

Tragically, the insidious cancer returned, and within five weeks of the book launch, she was gone.

During our last visit, as we were discussing her writing projects, that determination and defiance she was so well known for shone through one last time. Pondering her works in progress, she declared, "What am I doing lazing around in this hospital bed? I've got work to do!"

Thankfully, Helena never retired from her passions in life. She continued to teach at Vancouver Island University as a nursing professor until her death and she never stopped writing.

The determination, resourcefulness and courage of this woman will forever inspire those of us who knew her. To those of you who didn't know her, you will – very soon – when you turn the page.

— Peggy Grigor, Ladysmith Writers' Circle

The
Green Lady

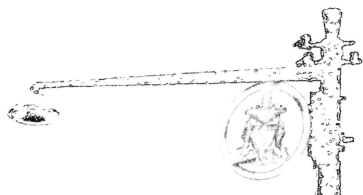

Chapter 1
Jean

The ringing stopped! The black earpiece felt icy cold as she recited, in an automatic voice, the seven digit telephone number. She was tired and weary following her long day, and craved sleep. Her patience was threadbare and her emotions drained from the constant tugging and pulling of the deprived human condition. The distinctive bakelite odour filled her nostrils with each deep and heavy breath as she struggled from deep sleep to brain alert. She swung her legs from the heat of the blanket nest and her feet automatically searched for the comforting lining of her sheepskin slippers.

"Who's phoning at 1:00 a.m.?"

Such was the lot of a domiciliary midwife! Who could it be? Perhaps Maisie McCall, with her three day-old twins? Or Jean Rennie in labour? These were the two women uppermost in Nell's conscious mind at that moment.

What a handful Maisie has, thought Nell, but she is a gritty wee thing and will manage her seven children eventually, despite that big waster of a man of hers. It is just that right now she needs a bit of help.

The pot of ham bone soup that Nell had put together on the coal fire range would have fed the older McCalls last night, but it was the twins that worried Nell. Maisie's milk was not in yet, and it should be, with the two wee hungry Horaces nuzzling away at her. Nell had taken in some free samples of baby milk powder for complimentary feeds for them. These babies needed extra feeding, as they looked as if they had lost weight before they were born; the wrinkled skin, the wizened look, and the fractious cries were all clues. It all added up.

The jangling of the pennies as they clattered into the metal mechanics of the phone box when button "A" was pushed, brought Nell swiftly to the present and with pencil in hand to the ready.

She said, "Sister Dickson here." It was Jean Rennie's husband, Alex, who spoke in a gruff voice. Maisie must be doing okay with her twins then, thought Nell.

"Sister, Jean's waters have broken in the toilet and she has pains, they started about midnight."

"Okay Alex, I will be there soon…" Nell replied, "…just encourage Jean to breathe the way I showed you."

"Okay sister, I'll do that but she is in a lot of pain!" Nell smiled at the sound of Alex's anxious voice, which was typical of most expectant dads.

"I'll be there as soon as I can", Nell reassured him, as she put down the phone.

She then immediately dialed the central office to let them know who was in labour and that she needed a corporation car and a gas and air machine. The car would pick Nell up and take her to the Rennie's home. She wondered about the Rennie's own home phone and why Alex had phoned from a call box? They were among a few of her patients who had a home phone, although it was a party line, which meant they shared the line with another family. Often, if the phone in one home was off the hook, the other party could not use theirs.

Nell was in motion and moved out of the bedroom. She was always afraid that she might slip back into the coziness of the bed and fall asleep. So at last Jean was in labour. It always amused her how the details of the "broken waters" were reported:

"Sister, mammy's water broke in the butcher shop," or "in the City Bakery" or "in the picture house in the middle of the news reel!"

So Jean's bag of waters burst in the toilet. That's what Nell would have expected from Jean, who was a neat and tidy freak. Her fastidiousness, Nell thought, hinged a wee bit on the obsessive-compulsive, however; secretly Nell admired this, as her own tendencies leaned the other way.

This was a long awaited event for Jean and Alex Rennie. They had been married for twelve years and this was what was called a "precious baby". At 32 years of age Jean was termed "elderly" to be having her first baby. Due to her age, Jean should really be confined in hospital. Nell knew that

Jean was terrified of hospitals, resulting from a bad experience as a child, but Jean's doctor told her she could stay at home, as long as Nell was comfortable taking on her case.

When Jean was seven she had been admitted to Belvedere Hospital with a severe bout of Scarlet Fever. She was in hospital for eight weeks, and hated every minute of it. Scarlet Fever was a debilitating infectious disease. Infected children were in quarantine in a "fever hospital" and the parents, who had to wear long quarantine gowns when they visited, could only wave to their child through a glass window. It was traumatic and distressing for both the children and the parents. The plan was to stop the spread of the disease.

¤

Nell, on the other hand, had also been in Belvedere with Scarlet Fever, when she was only five years old. Apart from the injections in the top of her right leg, she loved it. In fact, she often wondered if the whole experience sowed the seed of nursing within her. Her elder sisters told the tale that when she finally came home from hospital they were quarrelling, as siblings do, and found Nell crying into a large navy blue 'Scotty dog' that her sister May had made for her homecoming. When her Mammy asked what was wrong, she said that she wanted to go back to hospital because they don't fight there! They all "oohed" and "ahhed" at her and told the story over and over again to all the adults who came to visit.

May had made the dog out of an old heavy woolen skirt and stuffed it with old ripped nylon stockings. Nell couldn't bring her toys home from the hospital as they were deemed "fomites" (infection carrying) and had to be burned.

Nell never tired of the constant activity on the ward; there was always something going on. Nell liked to help the nurses change the bed linen. She wasn't allowed out of bed at first, so the nurses would bring the pillows to her cot for her to put the pillowslips on and tuck in the ends, the way the nurses had shown her. The fresh smelling laundered pillowslips were firm and smooth. She could make some of them stand up on their own if she opened them up. The cot was the size of child's bed and Nell had never seen anything like it before. If some of the younger children became fretful, the nurses would sometimes put them into Nell's cot so she could amuse them.

Meal times were interesting too. First Nell would see the "dinner man" bring in the stainless steel containers of food to the ward kitchen while two nurses would go round to all the beds and put the feeding bibs on the children.

Nell had a huge bib that hung on the locker rail. She could reach through the bars of the cot and get it ready for the nurses. They would always praise her for doing this with a "what a great help you are Nell" or "good for you Nell", or "thanks, Nurse Nell."

The ward Sister would then appear with the food containers on a trolley and proceed to dish out the meal for each child. She then handed the plates to the nurses, who would take them to the individual children. Some of the little ones needed to be fed, and there were usually some tears over food that they did not recognize.

"Ah don't want nat," was a common chant at meal time, but others, like Nell, ate everything and of course, the nurses reinforced this desired behaviour. The children in the ward had names for all the people that came to the ward. The bread deliveryman, who came at breakfast time, was the "bread man", the man who put down the mousetraps was the "mouse man" and there was the laundry man, the light man, the bin man etc.

Nell especially loved the evening time when the green shaded night light was lowered in the middle of the ward where the night nurses sat at the center cabinet. When the night nurse got up to answer a patient call, the light threw huge shadows as the nurse went to and fro about her business. The glow of the light was a comfort to Nell and seemed to her, to cast a magical spell over the ward. She liked the quietness, and the dimmed diffused light. She was now used to this darkness and wasn't afraid as she could always see a nurse. The nurses carried a torch, which created a white circle of light on the highly polished wooden ward floors, and wore their capes at night, which added to the magical scene. It was as if they floated around the ward, above the bright circle of light, with their white starched "Sister Dora" caps dotting above them.

There was a light outside the ward that shone in the window nearest Nell's cot and outlined the branches of an oak tree on the opposite wall. Even when the nurses pulled the blinds down, little chinks of the tree still appeared, and Nell would lie and look backward so she could see the rest of the branches dark silhouette against the beige paper blind. When the blind had not been pulled down, she could see the outline of part of the next ward's roof, as well as the sky. If it was a clear night, she could see some stars and perhaps the moon.

The time came for Nell and her hospital pal, Pam (another girl of five), to be up for a part of the day and they were taken into a large bathroom and dressed up in hospital clothes: white cotton sleeved vests and white liberty bodice with suspenders that buttoned on. There were also navy knickers with a pocket on the right knickers leg where you keep a hanky, and any other treasure you may have. Black thick "Lyle" stockings held up by suspenders and elasticized knickers legs came down over the top of the stockings, so that none of the leg was bare. There was black leather lacing-shoes with thick spongy soles, "like the nurse's shoes", Nell thought, to be tried on until a pair would finally fit. Nell was glad that her sisters had taught her to tie her laces. She tried to teach Pam to do it.

"Make a bunny's ear and go round the bunny's ear and through to make a second bunny's ear". They had to abandon the lace tying after many futile attempts.

The girls wore black woolen jumpers with collars that had three red stripes at the end. Over this attire they donned a navy gym tunic with a red sash that completed the outfit. It took time and effort to sift through the box labeled "girls age five to seven", to get the cape just like the nurses wore. These were made of black wool with flaming red flannel lining and black crossover straps, which fastened at the back of the waist.

Nell just adored this cape and experimented with it. She could hold the inside seams and pull it tight about her body or slip her hands through the hand slots and button the front, or leave the buttons open and let the cape fly behind her, held by the cross-over straps. The hood too was a wonder to her. So cozy, with the distinctive pleasant odor of wool encompassing her head.

The two nurses, Nurse Smith and Nurse McGinty, put their capes on and took Nell and Pam by the hand and escorted the two girls for a walk around the hospital grounds. They explained that they had to make their legs stronger before they could go home to their families. Nell enjoyed the attention and listened intently to the nurses chatting about their nights out at the Denniston Palais or the Lacarno, dancing, and nearly missing the last bus home:

"The big drip" that kept asking one nurse to dance and spoiling her chances with the heartthrob sailor. "The "old bitch of a night superintendent", who reported Nurse Smith for drinking a cup of tea on the ward, were among other juicy gossip! It was a good thing that the "old bitch" had not discovered Nurse McGinty having a sleep on a shelf in the linen cupboard, or the ball would have been on the slates then!

Nell had worked out that a "drip" had to be avoided and that a "heart throb" was to be sought after, from the non-verbal expressions and giggles of the two nurses. She also tried in vain to keep awake at nights to get a glimpse of the "old bitch", who Nell thought must look like an old witch and she wondered why Nurse McGinty slept in the linen cupboard with a ball!

Nothing much had changed about the nursing hierarchy when Nell did her training. Or had it? She remembered one night shift after the night superintendent did her rounds at two in the morning. She brought down a tea tray for herself and the other two nurses to the center cabinet, when like a puff, there was the Night Supervisor against the door of the large thirty-two bed "Nightingale" ward.

"Nurse Dickson, how many empty beds have you left?" asked Sister Scott.

"Three, sister, but one is an abortion bed," she replied. The surgical ward had eight beds for emergency gynecological complaints, which were known as the abortion beds. Sister Scott wrote down the information and smiled at Nell.

"Thanks, Nurse Dickson," and she vanished silently into the darkened hallway.

Sister Scott's smile reminded Nell of the time when, on Nell's first night duty as a junior nurse, she had come to Nell's aid with a young girl who aborted in the bed as Nell was in the process of admitting her. Nell's senior nurse was busy with a patient who had just returned from the Operating Theatre. Nell pushed the call bell and Sister Scott miraculously appeared and mentored Nell through the ordeal. Nell had been upset as the foetus, at sixteen weeks gestation, had some movement of its arms and legs and Nell thought that she had killed it by not knowing what to do. Sister Scott had reassured her that the foetus was not viable with life outside the womb at that gestation, and there was nothing that Nell could have done to save it.

Junior nurses were often in situations where they did not have the depth of knowledge in the subject matter and relied on the more senior nurses to make the decisions and give them the explanations. The "apprentice model", as it was called, could create a wonderful situated learning environment, or could be a great deterrent. There was learning by fire and then there was learning by being thrown into the inferno! In Nell's case, she decided then and there that she would like to learn more.

¤

Nell often thought that the only reason she was accepted into nursing training was that she was strong and healthy looking. It was a tough upward road they traveled. Thirty-two fellow classmates started in the "Preliminary Training School" (PTS) with Nell and only nine remained at the end of the three years of training. Nell then went on to do Midwifery training, which was another year. She liked being a midwife; it seemed to be part of who she was and became a way of life. She had a midwife's outlook on everything, just like a popular joke at the time: how does a midwife describe Winston Churchill? Great man, father of four!

Nell had booked Jean Rennie for a home confinement with the clear understanding that if Nell wanted her to go into hospital at any time during the labour, there would be no argument from Jean. Jean agreed to Nell's terms.

Jean Rennie was a librarian, employed by the world famous Mitchell Library at Charring Cross in Glasgow. She had read all there was to read on infertility and pregnancy. After all, she had the biggest reference library in Europe at her fingertips. They had been trying for a baby for the past eight years. Nell often wondered if the infertility had something to do with performing the "sex act" by the book, instead of just making love. She mused at the idea of Jean lying there on her back reading out the instructions to Alex, blow by blow (so to speak). But somehow, along the way the miracle happened and Jean was now pregnant.

On their first meeting, Jean had told Nell of the infertility problem.

"Sister, we tried everything; in the bed, out of the bed and up against the wall. We were getting all kinds of advice from all sorts of people, even people we hardly knew!"

Jean explained, "One day my friend Betty, who comes to my sewing bee, swore she became pregnant each time by taking a specific brand of cough syrup at night to relax her. So she brought me some, and 'bingo,' it worked."

Nell was amazed at the way Jean was so candid with her on their first meeting. But then so many women had great faith in the Green Ladies.

The Glasgow Corporation Midwives and Health Visitors earned the title because of the bottle green uniforms they wore: the green gabardine raincoats in the summer and the heavy green wool nap double breasted coat in the winter. The coats had large patch pockets and a buckled belt and the winter coat seemed to weigh a ton. Nell bought a green nylon raincoat to wear over the winter coat to save it from the rain, because it weighted two tons if it got wet! They also wore a brimmed felt hat in the summer and heavier velour hat in the winter.

Nell was nodding her head as Jean told her story and she tried to divert Jean's conversation away from the "old wives tales" of infertility remedies and all the positions the she and Alex had adopted.

Instead, she questioned Jean, "I hope you are not still taking the cough syrup, are you?"

"Oh no Sister, I read that you should not take any medication during pregnancy."

"That's great advice Jean," said Nell, feeling relieved.

Nell was thinking of the thalidomide case that was being researched at the moment. She did not want to talk about it to Jean and cause her anxiety, but was pleased that Jean would not take any medication without her doctor's approval. The thalidomide was, however, doctor prescribed. Nell had seen two affected babies when she was finished her Midwifery training and remembered the young resident doctor taking a full history on all the medications that the mother had taken during pregnancy. One of the mothers had not been prescribed the drug, but her friend had some that the doctor had given her. She had only taken one tablet, but her baby was badly affected.

Nell's first visit to Jean and Alex's home was in the evening, as Jean was still working during the day at that time. It was a cozy home and had all electric power. This was a modern trend initiated by the Government's Clean Air Act. Certainly, the Glasgow air was grossly polluted from all the smoke and grit from the heavy engineering industries found all over Glasgow. It was a busy industrial city and an important seaport, with shipbuilding along its famous River Clyde. When the fog fell it was not just misty, but all the grit and smoke would descend with it. The people called it "smog," a combination of smoke and fog. It was common to hear a passerby quip, "It's a right 'pea souper' the night". The smog left black sooty residue in the nostrils, and the bottom of Nell's nylon underskirts would become grey with the smog that would not wash out. People with respiratory ailments suffered greatly as a result of the smog, so it was a good idea to clean up the air.

The smog cut the visibility down to almost zero. Nell remembered being on a bus that was following the taillights of the car in front of it, and the bus turned into the driveway of the house! To be in the midst of it was really disorienting. When the smog cleared, there were abandoned vehicles everywhere. Smog masks were available. They were cotton filters to place over the nose and mouth and were held in place by a light aluminum frame that could mould round the nose and mouth. It shocked Nell to see the black soot that was trapped by the mask in such a short time. The smog always fell, of course, when it was icy cold and this added to the discomfort. Everyone bundled up with scarves wound around their heads and necks like balaclavas, trying to keep the cold and soot out, while leaving a slit for their peering eyes to register anything that loomed out of the depth of the smog. Shapes that suddenly appeared could be spooky and unnerving.

Coping with the smog was exhausting, as all the senses were on full alert. When Nell would arrive home, out of the smog, she would always have a hot bath and get rid of the soot particles. Home comforts were always much appreciated. The roaring fire and a plate of home made barley soup put things right, although her eyes would smart for hours after. Nell was always leery that she would get called out on a smoggy night. It made sense to clean up the air. The city plan was to make the center of Glasgow a smokeless corridor through the city in the direction of the prevailing winds. The first suburban smokeless zone was Pollokshaws with Pollokshields following in October 1961. It would not get rid of the fog and mist but would certainly reduce the smog.

Smokeless zones had their drawbacks too. Much of the household waste was usually burned on an open coal fire and more importantly to the midwife; the placenta was burned on the fire before the midwife left the home. However, other arrangements were made to take the package to the nearest hospital to be burned in the hospital incinerator. Nell was a known face at the Victoria Infirmary "boiler house", on her way home from a home birth.

Another alternative for citizens was to burn smokeless fuel. This was usually coal that had been processed and looked like charcoal. It burned at a higher temperature and caused no end of problems, necessitating the installation of new stainless steel back boilers, etc. There are always repercussions with any change that is made in society for the common good.

Jean had chosen electric off-peak storage heaters and electric fires for backup. The storage heaters used the electricity when it was at a lower tariff (usually during the night) and gave out the heat during the day.

Jean showed Nell the baby's room and the layette she had ready. This was going to be a well cared for baby. Nell loved to see the preparation that had been done and hear the mother's expectations around what they would and wouldn't do. Then, in the first few weeks of round-the-clock parenthood, the tiny baby taught them so much. She loved to see the transition and how quickly mother knew the child's different cries.

Jean and Alex's parents were being very generous too, as it was the first grandchild on both sides. Nell thought there was a wee bit of competition.

The high pram and cot had been picked out for the respective grandparents to buy when the baby was safely delivered. This was common practice among the Glasgow folks. You did not tempt providence: "Don't count your chickens before they hatch!"

Jean was a complex woman. She had many talents and had made long baby gowns from remnants of soft warm viella that she had acquired from a mill shop in Paisley. It was the custom to have the baby in gowns for the first six weeks before shortening them into baby clothes. The little all-in-one sleeping suits were available, but did not catch on as quickly as the tradition of the baby gown, which was seen as a birthright. The baby gown, matinee jacket, bootees, mitts and the woolen shawl were the way to go and the attire was simpler than it had been in the last decade. Babies wrapped in a woolen shawl had such a cuddly soft feel to them and they must have felt comfortable too.

When Nell did the first part of her midwifery training in the Rankin Memorial Hospital in Greenock, the babies were dressed in vests, muslin and terry nappy in a triangle shape. Another terry nappy was folded oblong and wound round like a kilt, as they did not use plastic pants on newborns. The next item of clothing was a barrycoat, which had a bodice and a flowing skirt that wrapped round the baby and tied at the waist. A long gown was put on over that and finally, a triangular flannel wrap, which kept the baby's arms in and prevented the baby from scratching their faces. The baby was then wrapped in a blanket and taken out to the mother for feeding.

The laundry generated by the nursery was colossal. During Nell's time here, a new matron came and changed a lot of things. The barrycoats went and the second terry nappy was replaced by a triangle of plastic. It was thought that plastic pants caused nappy rash, so the old fashioned ways were slow to go. In the islands, they used old pieces of woolen blankets round the nappy. Nell's father called the whole nappy thing "hipping": "The wean needs a hipping change," he would say!

The new matron also introduced rooming the babies in with their mothers. This change was hastened by the fact that part of a ceiling fell down moments after two nurses had passed with a patient trolley with nine babies on it, all lying like sardines across it en route for the ward. The sixties saw many changes in health care; it was the era for the movers and shakers in nursing to make their mark. What used to be done and what was done now was changing day by day and many were for the good, Nell

Jean

thought.

The corporation car drew to a halt in the Rennie's red chip driveway in Pollokshields. It was nice not to have stairs to climb for a change. Jean and Alex had bought the lower part of a divided villa. It was a large blonde-sandstone three-storied house with three attic dormer windows to the front and a small turret at one corner, giving the roofline an air of intrigue. The house was impressive and stood in its own grounds with large flat front and back gardens.

Nell entered and found Jean kneeling on the floor in a distressed state, with her head thrust into a pillow on the seat of an easy chair. Each of her hands grasped at the chair arms and Nell could see the scratch marks from Jean's nails on the uncut Marquette fabric. Her toes were in spasm, stretching and curling up in recoil, in a vain attempt to dissipate the pain.

Nell set to work to assess her stage of labour. She took Jean to the bedroom and helped her into bed. The labour pains were coming fast and furious and Jean's cervix was only two finger breadths dilated. This is going to be a long night if this was a posterior position, which Nell suspected, from the palpation and the fact that Jean's waters had broken before the labour pains began. The baby's heartbeat was good, so that was a positive. Nell talked to Jean and reassured her that everything was normal and she just had to take one contraction at a time.

Jean began to relax a little in Nell's presence. Pain did strange things to people; the quietest soul could turn into a raging bull in the presence of pain. Jean laboured on through the night with Nell at her side and Alex kept them company too, making sure that nourishment was at hand when needed. He also helped with the labour coaching. Nell relieved him when she saw that he needed a break. At seven fifteen, a baby girl entered the world.

"Is she like the world, Sister?" Jean asked, as Nell was guiding Alex to cut the cord.

"Yes," said Nell. "She appears to have everything that she should have."

The baby let out a cry as if to re-affirm Nell's statement.

"Have you decided on a name yet?" Nell inquired.

"Lorraine, I think," said Jean.

"We will put Margaret in for my mother and Helen in for Alex's mother."

"I have Helen in my name too," said Nell and added, "she could get Lorrie Peggy Nelly!"

They all laughed out loud, more from relief than the play on names. The afterbirth took 40 minutes to deliver. Nell was relieved and was pleased with the way things had gone for Jean. It had been a tough time and she had given Jean as much Pethidine for pain relief as she could and it did work a treat. Jean had used the gas and air machine during the transition stage, just to take the edge off the contractions.

There were a few times when Nell was on the verge of taking Jean into the hospital, but the baby's head rotated and progress was made. Nell always knew that if the waters broke before the pain started, it was usually a back labour and did take longer. But this baby must have read the book. After all, she did spend a good portion of her foetal life in a huge reference library! The baby took the shortened version of the posterior labour and turned sunny side up! Lorraine M. H. Rennie came looking upwards. Nell said that she would be a wee optimist! Nell did have to give Jean a few stitches.

"Can't be helped with this type of delivery, as the baby's head is born with the face looking upwards," she explained to Jean.

The first baby that Nell had ever delivered as a student midwife in the Rankin Memorial Hospital in Greenock was a face to pubis (sunny side-up). Nell remembered the sister midwife instructing her to increase flexion on the baby's head as it pushed against her left hand during the process of birth, but it seemed uncontrollable. Nell was shocked as she felt lumps and bumps under her hand. Her first thought was that the baby was abnormal, but the sister soon realized the situation and calmly said, "we have a baby looking up in the world." What a relief for Nell. This situation was the focus of talk among the student midwives that day.

It was close to eight in the morning when Nell bathed the baby. Alex opened the huge velvet drapes in the bedroom and let in a low wintry sun. The bedroom was large and had fourteen foot high ceilings, similar to all the rooms in this house.

The electric convection heating had kept the room at a steady temperature, making it comfortable to move around in. So often, with the coal fires in these big rooms, the area around the fire was warm, but if you wanted something from the other end of the room, it was cool! Peoples' fronts, facing the fire, could become toasty and their backs could be cold to the touch. Women who sat in front of the fires for long periods of time could end up with "corned beef tartan legs." This was what the Glasgow folks called the mottling of the legs, from the persistent radiant heat of the fire.

Glasgow expressions are wonderful, deep, multidimensional descriptions that cannot easily be translated into English or any other language. Glasgow humour is a quick wit that makes one smile at the drop of a hat, even though what the Glasgow folk had to smile about was a mystery to Nell. Perhaps it was some form of black humour, or just resilience against odds.

Jean's "Moses basket" on wheels, had been a family heirloom and passed around to all the babies in the Steel family (Jean's family). Each time it was used it was given a new coat of paint. This time a lead free paint was used. There was great hype about the level of lead in household paint affecting the health of children. Lead water pipes were being replaced with copper pipes.

Lead pipes were said to be "plumbo solvent" and allowed small amounts of lead to seep into the drinking water. Alex and Jean had replaced all the pipes in their place. Nell made them laugh when she told them that they had done the same in her apartment in Shawlands and that she had given the bin-men half a crown to take the lead pipes away! No wonder they always gave her a wave when they saw her. They probably made a fortune at the scrap yard! There was a big push on to rid the homes of lead cold water pipes.

Glasgow's water supply was hailed as being the best in Britain. It was a soft water, which came from the Barrhead catchment area of Loch Katrine via Milngavie. Milngavie is pronounced "milguy". Nell was familiar with the name as, when she was a child, if she burst into tears her father would say, "Oh there goes the Milngavie waterworks again!" Another Glasgow expression!

"You're just a wee cherub," Nell said, using one of her expressions for a time like this, and she meant it.

This baby had a shock of black hair that was sticking up as if the baby had a fright. She had a little rosebud mouth and her eyes were wide with an all-knowing expression.

Nell tended to the cord; one extra ligature on the stump of the cord round which she had a swab of surgical spirit, then placed the cord dressing round it. Then she sprinkled some special cord powder over it, folded the dressing neatly and secured it with a couple of turns of a crepe bandage around the baby's body; that was how the cord was dealt with. The baby looked like a wee doll when Nell had finished dressing her and put her in bed beside mum for heat and cuddles.

Alex had arranged to take a week of his holidays at this time and the two grannies would be over soon. Jean would be well cared for. Nell left to do her morning visits and would call back in to see Jean later. Nell would enjoy the transformation of Jean and Alex as they learned the ropes of parenting. She was pleased for the Rennie family.

Nell buttoned her double-breasted coat, slid the green belt through the green bakelite buckle and tugged to tighten it. Not unlike the marionette's strings, Nell collected herself together in mind, body and soul, lifted her case and was on her way.

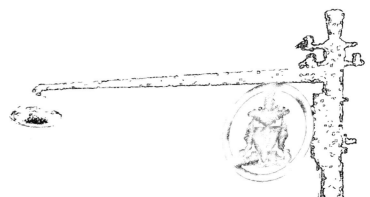

Chapter 2
Nell

Nell was born and World War Two broke out! Just before Nell's debut, the midwife hung her cardigan over the bedroom door handle to prevent her older sisters from looking through the keyhole. They were home from school at the lunch break and Nell arrived in time for lunch, so her three older sisters went back to school with the good news. Nell was the fourth girl in the family and was supposed to be the last try for the wanted boy.

When she first held Nell, her mother said to her, "Joy, joy, I wish you were a boy." When Nell was able to understand that story, she felt that she had been a disappointment from the day she was born. She was the fourth of five girls (no boys) born to Fanny and Bill Taylor. Her sister Agnes was born four years later and surprised everyone.

Nell, the disappointment, and Agnes, the mistake, grew up in wartime and post war conditions in Glasgow. This was a time of constant shortages of commodities. The black market was rampant, prefabricated houses were thrown up, the utility mark on goods represented an inferior quality and children were encouraged to drink concentrated orange juice which, after the war, was discovered to cause tooth decay! Ration books were necessary for the staples of life. From what Nell and Agnes could gather, if something was "pre-war" it was worth having. They loved to boast that they had dolls that were pre-war and they thought that their older sisters were special, as they knew more about pre-war stuff.

"The head, the legs and the arms of this doll are pre-war; you can see from the colour of its hair," Nell would say.

"How do you know that?" the pal would say.

"Because ma big sister got it from Santa before the war came."

"Oh that's dead good, can Ah play with it?"

"OK but don't break it or she'll kill me."

The Taylor family experienced a severe loss when their mother died at the age of thirty-six, following a cerebral thrombosis, then kidney failure. She suffered from a rheumatic heart that had resulted from many bouts of rheumatic fever as a child. A rheumatic heart is an enlarged heart: she had a big heart for people too. She was liked by everyone and was generous to a fault. One of Nell's earliest memories was her mother making ham and eggs for the bleach man, who was sitting in her house with a tartan rug round him.

The bleach man sold bleach door to door. He had a bicycle with an attached homemade wooden cart to hold the bottles of bleach. One day he had a mishap: something got stuck in the cartwheel and he took a tumble off his bicycle. He continued to sell door to door but when he got to the Taylor's door, Fanny noticed that he was quite shaken. He had a graze on his forehead, his trousers were ripped at the knee and the heels of both hands had gravel rash and dried blood on them.

"In the name o' the wee man, what has happened to you?" Fanny asked.

"Ah took a tumble off ma bike just at the corner there."

"Oh come away in…" Fanny replied, "…bring your bike into the close there…it will be quite safe. Here's a tartan rug. Now go into the bathroom and give me your breeks and I'll fix them up for you and get rid of the gravel on your hands. There's a nailbrush in there and you'll find TCP on the windowsill and a tin of Germoline cream should be there too. I'll make you a wee cup o' tea to steady your nerves."

"Mrs. Taylor you don't have tae dae this, you're busy with the weans," protested the bleach man.

"Dinna fash yourself, it won't take a jiffy," replied Fanny.

"Well if you are really sure…that would be a great help."

The bleach man's story was a sad one and Fanny knew it. He was trying to make a living to support his sick wife and his two daughters. He had just recovered from Tuberculosis and his old job would not take him back, as it was heavy duty. So he thought he would try to make it on his own, and get exercise and fresh air into the bargain. He worked on a commission only basis. His wife was still in Mearns Kirk Hospital, recovering from Tuberculosis, so he was looking after his two daughters, who were eight and ten years old. After his bacon and eggs he felt more composed and went on his way. Nell remembered that after her mother died, the bleach man would always stop to talk to her and always said what a fine woman her mother had been.

Fanny was kind and even gave the rag women cups of tea or cold drinks in the hot weather. The rag women were women who usually worked in pairs and would come to the door to ask for any old clothes. They would give you a cup or saucer or a balloon for the old clothes. Then they would gather all the clothes up in an old sheet and swing the bundle over one shoulder with their basket of goodies over the other arm, and would "wauchle" (waddle) on to the next house.

They all appeared to Nell to be "wee women" as she was as tall, if not bigger, than all of them. Perhaps being wee was one of the qualifications to be a rag woman. Often they had an old pram to help carry the loads of clothes. Sometimes they worked in conjunction with a ragman who drove a horse and cart onto which they would load their spoils. The ragman, who always wore a "bunnet", would also have a bunch of balloons and sometimes a bugle on which he would play a catchy tune.

Often, he would cry, "Any old clothes…good prices paid!" He would also say to the kids, "His yir mammy any old claise, hen? Ah'll gie yi a balloon fur them" or "his yir daddy any auld jaikits son? Ah'll gie yi some chewing gum fur them."

There was many a useful item that exited homes without the parents' permission, just to possess a colourful balloon or some Chiclets of chewing gum. The ragmen or women would be overjoyed if you brought out woolen stuff. They must have received a better price for woolens. Nell remembered giving some clothes at the door and receiving two cups with a gold loop design round the rim. The rag woman told her it was "real rolled gold".

Nell had never heard about real rolled gold before, but it sounded wonderful. When she told her sisters about the real rolled gold, they laughed at her.

"Pull the other leg Nell, there's a bell on it!"

She felt quite deflated, as she thought that she had somehow improved the family fortune. The rag trade must have paid good money, as there were a few different ragmen who came around in the summer.

One would rattle two dinner plates together and shout, "Pull the blankets aff yir bed and come and see ma china."

The china he was referring to were plates with the rolled gold design on them. There was always great interest around the ragman and kids would hang off the cart and try and "cadge a hudgie" (a ride) on it. Children would bring out carrots or sugar cubes to feed the poor mangy horse.

Penilee was a new housing scheme and most of the houses had gardens. When there was a horse and cart in the neighbourhood, her father would send her out with a shovel to collect the horse's droppings and she had to put them on the rhubarb. She was always so self-conscious about doing this, and was terrified that she would see some of the boys in her class, in fear that they would make fun of her.

"Shoveled any good horse manure lately Nell?" asked one of the smart alec boys, in front of the whole class. She blushed deeply, a beet root colour, to the roots of her hair! She never did forgive that boy, but did manage to knock him down during a game of rounders. He knew that she was trying to get even with him and didn't make a fuss.

The ragmen's horses provided some summer entertainment, to say the least. Nell never saw her mother entertain the ragmen but the independent rag women and the occasional Gypsy were sure of a friendly word and a cuppa from her. The gypsy women would tell fortunes as well as sell clothes pegs and bric-a-brac. The fortune telling would cause a buzz among the women and a few would gather in Nell's house. The kitchen was where the fortunes were told, while the rest of the women waited in the living room.

Those who had had their fortune told would come back into the living room and spill the fortune beans.

Nell and Agnes would hear, "How could she have known that…isn't that amazing."

"Do you know whit she telt me?"

Heads would huddle together with a chorus of "OOs and OOHs" and the occasional "help ma kiltie!"

Nell and Agnes would strain to hear the rest. But there was always some spoilsport of a woman who would say, "not for young ears," and point their finger repeatedly towards Agnes, Nell and their friends.

The fortune telling would culminate in the inevitable cup of tea and newly made treacle scones. Fanny could whip up treacle scones while she was talking to her friends. After the tea, Fanny would read the tea leaves left in the teacup, to much joviality. Fanny, being the perpetual optimist, would only read fortune!

The Taylor girls were devastated by the death of their mother. They had all seen her fall when the cerebral thrombosis happened. She was filling the kettle with water at the kitchen sink. The girls were all at the tea table and Nell remembered that there was a big bunch of bananas in the middle of the table. The kettle fell to the floor splashing water everywhere and her mother slumped to the floor. There were screams and tears and much confusion.

"Oh Mammy, Mammy, Mammy! Oh help, help, help!"

Someone ran for help. Someone put a pillow under Fanny's head. The paralysis was on her left side, so she was still able to speak. She was carried upstairs and the doctor was called. Nell was standing at the foot of the bed and Agnes was sitting on the bed with Fanny's right arm round her. Nell was smiling, as she did not know what else to do. Her older sisters were busy doing things that had to be done. The house had to be shining if the doctor was calling.

The last words Nell remembered her mother saying to her were, "And what are you smiling about, smiler."

"Ah don't know Mammy," was the reply.

Arrangements were made to transfer Fanny to Stobhill Hospital, which was at the other end of Glasgow from Penilee. As the ambulance men carried her down the stairs she was teasing them about their small stature and having to carry a stout woman like her.

"You lads will need to eat more for this job. You'll buckle at the knees under the weight of a big woman like me!" Fanny joked with the ambulance men.

"Not to worry…we've carried heavier folk than you, Mrs. Taylor."

Wee Agnes instinctively scurried out of the way as the ambulance men descended the stairs, as it was a tight bend towards the door. The girls looked on in disbelief.

"Don't worry, I'll be OK soon," Fanny said, as she was carried into the ambulance.

Stunned, they watched as the ambulance took their mother away. It disappeared round a corner and then they glimpsed it again, in the distance, as it tiered up the hill along Gladsmuir Road.

They did worry, and she died some weeks later, days before her thirty-seventh birthday. It was also a month before Agnes' fourth birthday and Eve's, (the eldest) seventeenth. Bill Taylor was left with five motherless daughters, a broken heart, a grudge against society, a strict work ethic and a volatile temper. Ten years later he did remarry. The family remained close; a case of together we stand, divided we fall.

The Taylor's were not a rich family but they were not poor either. They were a working class family in post war Britain. Bill was never out of work, so there was always steady money coming in each week and with all six mouths to feed, there was a steady stream of money going out each week. Trying to get ahead was a constant battle.

Mr. Taylor was adamant that good food was the only protection against illness. The big scourge of the times was Tuberculosis and he was afraid the girls would become infected. Good food and education were his priorities for the family. Wilma went all the way to Glasgow University and graduated with a Master of Art's Degree, MA, in 1957. She was the talk of the neighbourhood. People were pleased for her achievement.

One neighbour said to Bill, "Was it a BSA that Wilma got?"

He answered, "Aye and she got a 'Sturmey Archer' too!"

He laughed at that for years. Whenever there was a party and reminiscing would start, that was sure to come up in the conversation and Nell was amazed that it always evoked a hearty round of laughter. A BSA was a bike and a "Sturmey Archer" was a special gear system for the bike!

House parties were a highlight of Nell's childhood and she wished her father could always be as happy as he appeared when a party was in full swing. The New Year parties were always a hit and family or friends visiting would turn into a "gay and hearty" when Bill would play his fiddle. Eve would play the piano and a good old singsong round the piano always erupted. After all the Scottish songs were exhausted, on came the Irish songs. Bill liked to sing about Paddy McGloan. Nell learned the words, which did puzzle her when she was young.

> *Oh! Paddy McGloan forgot that he was dead, dead, dead*
> *He rose up in his coffin and he said, said, said*
> *"If this wake goes on one minnit*
> *The corpse he must be in it*
> *You'll have to fill me drunk*
> *To keep me dead."*

Bill was a widower for ten years and he remarried the year Nell began her nursing training in the Southern General Hospital. Bill did not want any of his daughters to be nurses. He would not let May be a nurse because no daughter of his was going to be a "skivvy" and empty bloody bedpans.

Nell had her stepmother to thank for persuading him that it would be a good idea for Nell to go into training. She argued that with Nell gone, it would only leave May and Agnes at home, as Eve and Wilma were already married by this time.

It was her stepmother, Beth, who went with her to book in at the nurses' home on the eve of her starting date. Beth loved to tell the story that she had just arrived back home when Nell appeared at the door—she had forgotten to take the money for her text books—they thought that she had changed her mind about taking nursing!

Nell loved nursing overall, but there were tough times when she would have given up. However, when she could hear her father saying, "You'll never stick to it," she would do anything to prove him wrong. After her initial training, Nell went on to Greenock to the Rankin Memorial Hospital to do the first part of her midwifery training. A dear friend who had trained there inspired her to try it.

Nell would come back up to Glasgow on her days off or for an evening out, and as the train crossed the Clyde on its way into Central Station, Nell would have an involuntary gulp and a tear in her eye; she did love Glasgow. The train journey to Greenock only took twenty-five minutes!

Nell met her future husband in the Southern General Hospital. It was a nurse-patient romance. Scott Dickson was recovering from a bout of malaria and he was on a trial of new medication.

He would jokingly say, "I wasn't well when I met you, you took advantage of me!"

Scott was in the British armed forces in a special army detachment, which meant that he was away from home for long periods of time. They corresponded and met from time to time and were married two years later.

Nell Dickson was newly married when she accepted the post as Domiciliary Midwife for Glasgow Corporation. Scott only had three years to go in the armed forces before he would look for a civilian job, so this type of work suited Nell at this time. They had purchased a flat in Grantley Gardens in Shawlands. This was a suitable location, as it was between Pollokshaws Road and Kilmarnock Road, both of which were major bus routes that Nell came to rely on.

Domiciliary Midwifery was work that Nell loved. Yes, it was physically demanding, and being on call six nights a week was harrowing at times, but above all, it was a worthwhile occupation. At any one time, the district midwife knew everything that was going on in her geographic area, including how many babies were due to be born. Her partner–midwife worked in an adjoining area and they covered each other one half day, one night, and one whole day till midnight (and of course for holidays too).

Once per week, all the domiciliary midwives paid a visit to the head office at 112 Ingram Street in Glasgow, where they submitted their paper work and patient records. These entailed the prenatal records, labour and delivery or confinement records and postpartum records. There was also the notification of birth card to be filled out. All of these records needed to be meticulously completed.

The midwives also stocked up on their supplies at the office on Ingram St. They were allowed to prescribe and administer medications such as injectable narcotics, narcotic antidote, a "toco promoter" and vitamin K. These were all obtained from the head office pharmacist, who, along with the midwives themselves, kept a copy of medication records.

Another time the midwives met was at the monthly Royal College of Midwives meeting, which was usually held at Glasgow Royal Maternity Hospital. At these meetings Nell met other midwives from hospitals and from the district and there was usually an interesting speaker and a time to chat. The domiciliary midwives were, of course, on call, but were easily reached at this location.

Nell enjoyed the trips to the office on Thursdays. She met up with her colleagues from all over the city and there was a lot of shop talk. Four or five of them would go to the tearoom of Campbell, Stewart and MacDonalds, which was a department store warehouse open to members. They would order shortbread and Russian tea before making their way down to St. Enoch Square or along to Hope Street to catch a bus back to their respected areas. The Russian tea was served in a glass tumbler set in a silver holder with a handle. It was tea with lemon and had a silver plunger to squeeze out the lemon juice into the tea. Nell loved to see the tea lighten in colour as the lemon juice diffused into it when the plunger was depressed. The shortbread fingers complimented the tea perfectly. It was the best shortbread Nell had ever tasted.

Shortbread had another strong memory for Nell. She remembered many New Year Days when she and her young sister Agnes would come downstairs to find the remnants of the Hogmanay party. On the table there would be black buns, shortbread, bottles of homemade ginger and raspberry non-alcoholic wine. This wine had been made from the Co-op's "Yuletide essence". Just add boiled water and sugar and the wine could be bottled. Nell loved the throat burning taste of the ginger wine, softened by the butter smoothness of the shortbread. She did not care for the black bun. It always puzzled Nell why this wine was only made for Hogmanay. She supposed it was to keep it special.

There were lots of things that were only done for Hogmanay. Projects had to be completed before the New Year dawned, or they would never be finished. There would be a mad dash to get knitting or sewing finished before midnight so that the New Year would have a clean slate.

One year, when Nell was a student nurse, she was knitting a pullover for her father's Christmas present. She was on night duty and she thought, no sweat, there would be plenty time to finish the knitting. But there had been a flu epidemic and it had been too busy to knit, so she farmed parts of the pullover out to different nurses who had offered to help. What a disaster! All the tensions were different and the pullover looked terrible, but it was finally finished on the 30th December! She never saw her father ever wear it.

Nell loved Hogmanay. Everything in the house was cleaned. Even the ashes were lifted from the fire just before midnight so that the fire would burn bright to bring in the New Year. Everyone had a bath and washed their hair and put on new clothes to welcome the New Year. No one touched the eats or the drink till the bells of the New Year chimed. Then the doors and windows would be opened to let the Old Year out and the New Year in. The ships on the River Clyde would sound their foghorns and some churches would ring their bells. The churches near Nell held watch night services, just as they did for Christmas, so if you were so inclined, you could begin the year at church. Nell, with one of her student nurse friends, did this several times and it was memorable.

These were the days when the midwife, like the policeman, walked or rode on public transport. Only one or two of the midwives had a car. When Nell was called to a confinement, the Glasgow Corporation car collected the gas and air machine from the central depot and then collected the midwife from her home, then on to the woman's home. The midwife had two cases: one was a confinement case and the other a postnatal/prenatal case. These cases were metal and replaced the older styled leather doctors' case. They had been well designed. Inside, there were metal studs that held a linen liner. The linen liner had linen pockets and loops where the midwife placed her instruments on the inside of the lid. The main part of the case accommodated all the rest of her supplies. She had a good amount of these changeable liners. On the outside of the case was a navy blue gabardine (waterproof) cover, which had a large flap pocket on one side. The case had two locks and a metal handle.

The flap pocket was useful to carry maps, small change purse and diary with phone numbers—things that required easy access. One day Nell had bought some lamb's liver on the way home at lunchtime and popped the small package into the pocket of the case. She was hurrying to the bus stop, as she knew her bus would be along soon.

No sooner had she got to the bus stop when she heard a voice getting louder and louder calling, "Sister, Sister."

She turned round to see a boy of about seven years of age running towards her, calling as he ran, "Sister, Sister."

He seemed to be agitated and distressed and she turned to him, concerned for his state of alarm. He was dressed in a grey school uniform; grey short pants that came just below his knee and obviously bought for growth, his grey wool blazer flapping open to reveal a grey hand knitted V-neck sweater with black and red stripes round the neck. His white shirt sported a black and red school tie, loose at the collar, the would-be Windsor knot unraveling as he ran. His grey knee length socks were at half-mast, but he was fully intent on running at full speed in his black brogue shoes. His cap, complete with the school badge, managed to defy all laws of gravity and stayed on his head, although the skip was heading towards his right ear.

They were now within a couple of yards of each other and the boy blurted out, as he slowed his pace, "Oh Sister, the wean in yir bag is bleedin' an it's drippin' oot!"

Nell looked down at her case and sure enough, there was blood dripping from the pocket seam that had left a trail from the butcher's shop to the bus stop. She assured the boy that everything would be fine and thanked him for letting her know. Luckily, her bus drew up and saved the day as she waved and smiled to the boy through the window. Once seated, Nell, smiled to herself and, being careful not to stain anything, she slipped her plastic rain mate under her bag. She would have to give the cover a good scrubbing or she would have all the dogs in the area after her. Dog control in the City of Glasgow was often out of control. The dogs appeared to take the Glasgow motto to heart, "Let Glasgow Flourish," although the full motto reads:

*Oh Lord let Glasgow flourish
By the preaching of Thy word
And the praising of Thy name.*

Children really did think that the midwife brought the baby in the bag. Nell thought that this was kind of magical for young children and prolonged childhood, as soon enough the realities of the world would be on their shoulders. She remembered going to a confinement in Norfolk Street in the Gorbals district on the south side of the River Clyde. It was not one of her own patients, but the midwife for that area was already on a call. As the corporation car drew up at the close entrance, Nell stepped out of the car and reached for the gas and air case, but she found that her confinement case was being snatched out of her hand!

"Wait! What the Dickens?" she screamed, as she quickly turned round and found herself eye to eye with a boy of about fourteen.

He was holding the case as if it was made of fragile glass; one hand tightly holding on to the handle at his nose level and the other hand supporting the bottom of the case. Nell was desperately trying to make sense of this encounter.

Then a voice from behind the case said, "Sister ma mammy sent me tae help ye, I'll carry the wan wi the wean."

Here was this boy, who physiologically was old enough to father a child, still believing that the midwife brought the baby in her case. He was a tubby sort of a lad with black tousled hair and was wearing a red and white football strip (Clyde Football Club colours). The studs on his football boots made him look taller.

He continued, "Ma Mammy yelled from the windae when she saw the black cor,…you know wur in Sister,…it's right to the top."

"Yes! It would be the top flat." Nell often wondered if fertility had anything to do with living on the top floor!

Every one of her deliveries lately, seemed to be on the top floor! As she climbed the stairs behind him, she thought about how this big lad was going to feel very silly very soon, when he realized the true facts of life!

However, when Nell met his Mammy, she understood why the boy still believed that babies arrived in the midwives case, as whatever his Mammy said he believed. If she said babies came from the moon, then so be it! She was a force to be reckoned with! In all Nell's years being a domiciliary midwife she was never really afraid of any of the men that she met, but had a healthy regard for some of the women. There were a few that she would prefer to keep on their good side. They were all a product of life experiences and environment, hence the birth of the expression, "You can always tell a lass from Glasgow, but you can't tell her much!"

Too true, they were no-one's fool.

Nell's sister, Eve, worked in a shipping office in Glasgow. It was the White Star Line where she was a typist. She had the job of addressing return envelopes and when they would arrive back in the mail, she noticed more than one time that she had typed the "Shite Star line". She was in a panic, in case the battle-axe of an office manageress would find out about it. She would tell the family all about the office stories. One office girl from Gorbals was the center of many of the stories.

The office boys kept annoying her and trying to make her embarrassed, till she got a hold of one of them against a wall and said in a clear voice, "Any mair o' yir capers an Ah'll staple yir baws the-gither."

The point was well taken and she never had any bother again from the pranksters.

Nell was 23 years old and was, at that time, the youngest domiciliary midwife employed with the Glasgow Corporation. She worked with her partner-midwife who showed her the ropes, and Nell attended two confinements with her. Then she was on her own.

It was 4 a.m. when the car collected her from home and she was soon entering the once grand Victorian buildings in Abbotsford Place, in Glasgow's Gorbals. She had the gas and air equipment in one hand and her confinement case in the other. These had been beautiful apartments on Glasgow's south side that were now, sadly, in a sorry state of disrepair. The crumbling pieces of sandstone and society were falling side by side, grain by grain.

Nell often wondered what it had been like in its hay day. Many Jewish families had lived in this area before moving further south to Shawlands, Giffnock and Newton Mearns. She imagined the women with their long gowns and bustles, bustling to and from in this thriving community. By the lamplight, Nell could see the faded business plaques on the stonework as she entered the close: Dentist, Dressmaker, Corsetiere, Doctor and Jeweler, to name but a few. Still in existence, further down the street, was Geneen's restaurant, specializing in Jewish food.

Once through to the rear of the building, there were spiral stairs enclosed in cylindrical brick turrets that reminded Nell of castle-like structures. Luckily, the lights were on in the stairwell, as it could be very dark without the streetlights shining through the landing windows. It could be spooky too.

Nell knew a collection agent who got a real fright one evening in these buildings. He was climbing a set of stairs like these, in the pitch dark, and something hit him on the back of the head. He froze! He thought that his unlucky day had come and that he was being attacked. He lashed out with punches right, left and center but felt nothing except a cold feeling in his legs as he stumbled over his trousers, which he discovered round his ankles. His braces had burst with the weight of the money in his pockets and it was the back braces that had hit him in the head! He stood there and laughed and once he had wrapped the braces round the trousers like a belt, he called it a night.

Nell was glad that the lights were on as she climbed the stairs, searching each door she came to for the correct address, as this was an unknown patient to her. She was rehearsing in her mind all the things she would do for the set up. She wanted everything to be perfect.

This flat was huge and she entered through a wide open door into a large square dark hall. There was one lonely looking 40 watt bulb hanging from beautifully ornate center cornicing, trying its utmost to illuminate the space. The hall was void of furnishings and each of the huge six heavy paneled dark wood doors seemed to dim the bulb's efforts. All the rooms were sublet to different tenants and they had to share the kitchen for cooking. One door was ajar and a shaft of light shone from it into the hallway, like a beacon in a dark bleak night, outlining the silhouette of a lonely hunched figure on the floor scrubbing the lino. This was the labouring woman in the last stages of "nest making."

"Let me help you into the room Kate," said Nell, once she had deposited her cases. It didn't look as if there would be time for the big impressive set-up.

"OK," was the reply.

"How often are the pains coming?"

"All the time, it seems," said Kate.

"Lie up on the bed and I'll examine you so we can see what's what."

"OK, sister," Kate replied.

Kate removed a pair of gent's cotton underpants that she had been wearing and climbed on the bed complete with a black mini skirt and a pink polo-neck jumper. As Kate moved her legs apart, Nell could see the unmistakable perineal bulge of the baby's head.

"No need to examine you...the baby's head is just sitting there...a few pushes and you'll have this baby."

There was no reply from Kate. Luckily Nell was well prepared and she opened her case, pleased that all her anxiety had gone. She felt in control and proceeded to deliver a beautiful baby girl between the black knees and below the hiked-up mini-skirt! No fuss, no bother! Just a perfect, text book delivery. That was her initiation into domiciliary midwifery! The blacked-kneed woman coped silently with her labour just as she coped with the rest of the heartbreak in her meager, uncertain life.

Nell bathed the baby and tried to make conversation with the mother. Kate Sorley was the name she was using, but Nell's partner-midwife had cared for Kate some years before under another name. All her five children were in care and she was obviously on the run from something or someone. It is difficult to run with a newborn baby.

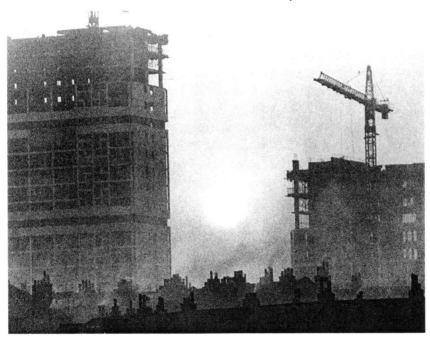

The other woman there was the landlady. She did not speak much either. There were, however, some new baby clothes to welcome this wee mite into the world. Nell silently planned to bring Kate some baby things that her friends kept giving her, things that Nell saved for such new mothers like Kate.

Her first independent confinement completed, Nell felt a surge of satisfaction and peace within herself. It suddenly dawned on her that she had achieved what she had worked hard to prepare for. She really was a Glasgow Domiciliary midwife! She so looked forward to an eventful career, full of interesting experiences and colourful characters.

Nell buttoned her double breasted coat, slipped the green belt through green bakelite buckle, tugged to tighten it, picked up her case and left, just as the dawn was breaking over the Gorbals.

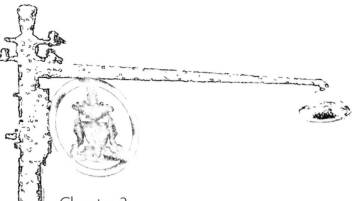

Chapter 3
Maisie McCall

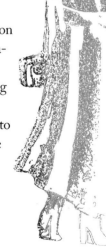

The morning bustle had begun, as Nell walked along Nithsdale Road. She would visit Maisie McCall first. She worried about the twins and their feeding; should they require a doctor to review them? She wanted to sort that out early in the day. Great! There was the bus she needed. Nell broke into a run towards the bus stop. The bus horn tooted and came to a halt beside her.

"Thanks a million," she called out to the driver, who tipped his green cap at her.

"Good morning, Sister," said the clippie, as Nell boarded the orange and green bus, "is it a good morning. Another wean in the world and like the world I hope?"

"That's right, a lovely wanted baby girl!" Nell smiled as she flopped onto the green leather seat, which was cool to the touch. The bus lurched forward and they were on their way.

Walking again, she passed many groups of children on their way to school. Nell loved the smatterings of conversations she heard as they passed by her:

"There's the baby Sister, she might have a wean in her bag the day."

"Tee hee hee," and they would giggle with their hands to their mouths, their shoulders slightly hunched and all the time watching Nell.

"It wis good at the brownie's last night so it wis."

"Ah didnae tell her, she would've kilt me!"

"Can you keep a secret?"

"Ah've goat toast fur ma play piece, whit huv you goat?"

"Oh Ah've goat two chipped apples to eat at play-time."

The chat amongst these youngsters always made Nell smile to herself.

Nell saw Shirley McCall hurrying down the road and called, "Hello Shirley!"

"Hello Sister. Are you goin in tae see ma mammy?" asked Shirley.

"Yes Shirley, that's where I'm heading for right now," replied Nell.

"Oh that's good; you'll cheer her up, Sister. She likes you, Sister. Ah'll need tae run or Ah'll be late. Ah was feedin' wee Douggie."

"You've still got ten minutes Shirley, bye."

Shirley ran off to school with her bag swinging over her shoulder and her mop of uncontrollable blonde curls bobbing about.

Nell knocked at the door, which was open slightly, and called, "It's Sister Dickson, Maisie."

"Oh come away in, Ah'm gled tae see ye Sister. I'll pour ye a cup o' tea. Shirley, the wee soul, baked fur me last night and, wonders will never cease, there's some scones left. Butter and jam OK?"

"Maisie I'll get it. You sit down and tell me how the babies have been feeding since six o'clock last night," Nell inquired.

The McCall twins were a lightweight for mature babies and needed feeding. Daniel, the eldest was 6 lb and Douglas was 5 lb, 5 oz. Although they were full term babies they were really wrinkled at birth, a fact that made Nell suspect a possible loss of weight before they were born. Maisie, in the past, had produced nine and ten pounders in spite of her 4 foot 10 stature.

Maisie loved to tell the story of her Obstetrician, at Glasgow Royal Maternity Hospital, which was affectionately known to the women of Glasgow as "Rotten Row," who she quoted as saying, "Maisie you amaze me, I think we could drive a corporation double-decker bus through that pelvis of yours!"

Maisie never had any trouble in the actual deliveries of her babies. The latest arrivals were bonnie babes, identical twins and had soft pale pink skin with flaming red hair and tempers to match, if the volume of the cry was an indicator!

Yes! thought Nell, wee Danny and Douggie McCall would be a challenge and a handful to rear. Maisie was exhausted though, as her pregnancy had not been without its problems The pre-eclampsia had occurred in the last trimester and the varicose veins, with their rope-like knots, made her constantly worry of phlebitis or worse.

The sheer physical effort of carrying twins and looking after her other five children, all under the age of nine, was debilitating and tiring, with little help from that big galoot, Hector, who insisted that his mother had ten weans and never missed a step! He failed to remind those listening to him that his mother died before she left her childbearing years. Nell had shared Maisie's prenatal care with the GP, Dr. Stone, and the specialist from Rotten Row. She had impressed on Maisie the importance of her going into Rotten Row for her confinement. Nell had delivered all five of Maisie's children but there could be unseen and unpredicted complications with a twin delivery. Maisie promised Nell that she would do that.

However, four nights earlier, at 3 a.m., Nell's phone had awakened her with that piercing ring.

Shirley, Maisie's eldest (who, incidentally, was named after Shirley Temple) was calling from the local phone box, summoning Nell with the usual cry, "Can you come quick Sister? Ma mammy needs you!"

When Nell got there, all was arranged for a home confinement. The fire was burning in the grate, a pot of water was boiling away waiting on the midwife's instruments, and the confinement box was to the ready as were the bottles of Dettol and Arachis oil. A brand new pair of bright yellow flannelette sheets, still in the packet, were placed near the fire. A hot water bottle was warming the middle fold of each sheet bundle. The new pair of "flanny sheets" was what many midwives requested the women should do with some of their home confinement grant money. Many of the women would take out a twenty-week ménage at a textile store and this would give them enough for sheets, towels, nappies and baby blankets.

The ménage was a great idea; twenty women would pay a decreed amount every week for twenty weeks and would all pick a number from one to twenty. Each number represented the week that each person could spend twenty times the payment. It was a good way of keeping out of debt and having ready cash to buy the extras. The flannelette sheet bundle made for a cozy bed for the newborn child against the ravaging cold of the Scottish weather, summer or winter! Later, it gave the family a pair of bed sheets. It made good sense when money was tight.

The scene was warm and bright, with the flickering of the coal fire throwing a homey glow over the surroundings. Two little vests, gowns, hand knitted cream-coloured matinee jackets, hats and bootees to match the jackets, all lined up on the fire guard, all ready with the towels and the baby bath. Many women whose pregnancy condition warranted a hospital confinement called the midwife at the last minute to avoid going into hospital. The reasons for doing this were varied, but the main one was that they did not want to be away from their home turf. They were the glue that held the family together and besides that, they held the strings of the family purse. Also, they received a Government home confinement grant if their baby was delivered at home!

¤

This was the early sixties and although the Prime Minister, Harold McMillan, said the people of Britain "never had it so good," for many families in Glasgow, life was a constant struggle to make ends meet. The post war housing schemes were thrown up in answer to the demand for more housing and little attention was paid to proper community planning, which led to long commutes for the people to reach employment, decent shopping, schooling and entertainment. People moved from the overcrowding of the inner city to the more spacious houses of the schemes, but they soon found that they felt alienated from their families and it was almost impossible to move back. Valium seemed to be the panacea to fight the blues of the housing schemes. It was not uncommon in the inner city to find whole families living within a stone's throw from each other. This type of family support was as strong as iron. The new houses lacked the warmth of the old tenements. Many had concrete floors—suitable for the Tropics but not for Glasgow's northerly climate, which shares the same latitude as Moscow!

¤

The McCall's place was usually warm, it was one of the older houses, and they always seemed to have enough coal, as Hector sent the three older boys along the side of the railway to collect the pieces of coal that fell off the train tenders. A wee handful of coal could keep the fire going for a good hour or so. Maisie also augmented the fuel with the use of coal briquettes and by burning the potato peelings wrapped in newspaper and covered by a shove full of coal dross. Old shoes were a stand by for a cold night as they gave off a great heat. Maisie was a great wee manager. Her Granny in Lanark had brought her up, and she could cook and bake without recipes, as well as knit and sew. There was always something on the stove and on the knitting needles.

Her mother and father had lived in Paisley and they both worked in the Paisley Thread Mills. Maisie was born in Paisley, but went to live with her Granny when her father joined the Royal Air force at the beginning of World War Two. He was killed in 1940. Her mother moved to Glasgow and worked as a waitress in the prestigious Rogano Restaurant. She had such unsociable hours of work, so it was deemed that Maisie had a more stable life with her Granny, and a safer one too. Children were often evacuated from the city when the German air raids on Glasgow and the Clyde-side shipyards were rampant. The Glasgow "blitz" ravaged the city and the Clyde side, right down to Greenock. Maisie was safer away from that devastation.

Maisie could feed her family with a pot of soup made from potato, whatever veggies she could find and a big marrowbone. Her children were the focus of her life. Tending to them was a full time job and she wanted to give them a mother's love first hand, providing the kind of closeness that she had missed with her own mother. She was certainly on good terms with her mother now, but felt that her mother was overwhelmed with all the bairns, as she was herself at times. Her mother was always on about Hector's lack of drive and it got tiresome listening to the constant barrage of insults towards him. Wartime did tend to mess-up many lives and leave scarred and bitter resentment deep within the soul.

Nell admired Maisie McCall for her sheer spunk and the ability to make her pennies stretch. Hector McCall, on the other hand, needed a swift kick in the backside to get him motivated. He couldn't keep a job and it did not seem to bother him if he was idle and, into the bargain, money ran through his fingers like water. He was a handsome big lad of six feet two, with a shock of carroty red hair and a face full of freckles. He had a broad smile that lit up his face and crinkled his eyes at the same time. His mother had come from the Gorbals and his father from Islay. His father was a marine engineer on the MacBrayne shipping line that serviced the Hebridean Islands. Mr. McCall senior was home every Friday night and away again on the Monday morning, so Hector was brought up mainly by his mother and his older sisters. There was always enough money in that McCall family and, as Hector was the youngest, he wanted for nothing.

Nell could not make up her mind if he was just plain daft or if he was really dead crafty. After their fifth baby was born, when Maisie had a severe hemorrhage from which she nearly died, Nell had talked to Hector about family planning. She had spelled it out in words of one syllable, drawn diagrams and told him of all the options. He fully agreed that five children were a lot of wee mouths to feed and growing bodies to clothe. He agreed too, that Maisie needed a break from being pregnant; she needed to regain her strength. Nell even made an appointment for him to go to Park Circus, to the Family Planning Clinic, to talk about him having a vasectomy. But, obviously he had not followed through on that course of action; probably spent the bus fair on a bet at the dog racing.

Here they were a year later; Maisie with a troublesome twin pregnancy and Hector with a bigger boast to his manhood that ever before, all because of the want of the bus fare and a wee bit of initiative. He wasn't a bad man, he just needed to grow up and face his responsibilities—all eight of them! Life was hard and reliable work difficult to find. The sociologists' slogan about children born in these depressed areas was "born to fail," but then, the sociologists had not met the women like wee Maisie McCall, who would fight for the rights of her children.

When Nell arrived at 3.30 a.m., four nights ago, Maisie was in the middle of the kitchen on her hands and knees, scrubbing the floor. Both hands were on the large brown scrubber, arms extended, and her head almost touching the linoleum that was covered with soap bubbles that blew about with each heavy breath that Maisie took during each labour pain. Many labouring women adopted this pose, as it helped distract them from the pain, and, at the same time, the position greatly eased the backache, prevented a drop in blood pressure and, of course, scrubbing the floor made the place clean and smell of washing soap for the new arrival.

Nell helped a somewhat wet Maisie to her feet. Two large, fierce looking mongrel dogs that had to come to offer their mistress some protection flanked them. Lassie and Rex shoved their wet noses in wherever there was a space between Nell and Maisie. Nell glanced at Lassie's eyes and was pleased to find that her eyes were clear. Last time she was here, Lassie had runny mucky-looking eyes, and after she had finished her visits for the day, she had gone back and treated the dog's eyes. A half-cup of cooled boiled water and the tip of a teaspoon of salt made a good saline solution and she bathed the dog's eyes with it. Then she instilled some erythromycin eye ointment from little applicaps, which were a one-dose and throw away type of deal. She kept some outdated applicaps for such occasions; the fresh ones were, of course, for the newborn baby's eyes, to prevent eye infections.

As the two women progressed toward the recessed bed in the kitchen, Nell watched Maisie's gait. Nell knew from her observations that Maisie was in second stage of labour and about to push. One of the older midwives from Gorbals had told Nell what to look for and it had proved right every time.

"If you see them on their tip toes and if the angle of their back is like this…" and she demonstrated the position, "…then they don't have long to go before they deliver."

Nell loved to listen to experienced midwives as they had such great tales to tell and had started to practice with much less back up than she had now.

"Maisie you should be in Rotten Row—you know what you promised," Nell said quietly.

"Aaw sister, I'm sorry, but that big buggar hasnae come hame yet from the dugs an Ah couldnae leave ma weans. He'll huv missed the last bus from the White City an it's a lang walk hame. The pains jist hit me all of a sudden a wee while ago. It'll be OK noo that your here, sure it wull? Shirley hen, get the Sister a wee cup o' tea wull ye? Oh Sister, Ah think Ah'm going to push."

The guttural sounds that emitted from Maisie sent Nell into a motion that was determined, calculated and calm. Nell examined Maisie to find that there was a little foot leading the first twin into the world. She also noticed that Maisie had two black knees where she had been kneeling on the floor.

Maisie's groans were low and determined, so Nell wasted no time in writing easily read instructions for Shirley to read to Dr. Stone over the phone. There was no time to get Maisie to hospital, perhaps a flying squad later, if there proved to be complications, but she needed Bill Stone here.

She gave Shirley three pennies for the phone and the note for Dr. Stone to come at once. She also told Shirley to take the Rex with her. He was a good part Alsatian and was very protective of the children. He also looked fierce! She hated like hell to send a girl of nine out in the middle of the night to walk a couple of streets away to the phone box, but what else could she do? She certainly couldn't leave at this stage.

Big stupid appearance! Hector should have been here. At least he could have done the phoning. Normally the doctor was only called for if there was a problem that was out with the midwife's scope of practice. Nell would normally call the doctors' surgery to let them know that their patients were labouring if it was during the day, or phone them in the evening as a matter of courtesy, but they only came out if there was a problem.

A twin delivery is inherent with potential problems. "Locked twins" was Nell's biggest fear with a home confinement. This occurs when the first baby is breech (as this one was) and the second twin's head traps its head and the chins lock in position. When this happens, one baby has to be destroyed to allow the other baby and the mother to live. From Nell's examination, the second twin appeared to be lying across Maisie's abdomen, but this could change at any minute.

She had not yet received a copy of the x-ray report from Rotten Row telling of the position of the babies and, of course, if Maisie was in hospital as arranged she could receive readily available intervention to avoid disaster. Nell remembered how Maisie had described the x-ray to her. "They lie ye doon oan yir stomach and pit a big belt oan ye so ye don't move. I felt as if Ah wis goannae burst! I wish they could see into your belly without strapping ye doon like that. That wis worse than labour!"

Little did Maisie know, at that very moment, Professor Ian Donald, an Obstetrician who was working at the other end of Glasgow, was pioneering ultrasound.

In her mind, Nell was reassessing all the factors at hand. Maisie had a good-sized pelvis, and that wee leg did not feel too chubby. Maisie was having good strong contractions, so that was another positive. Dr. Stone would come out, as she knew he was on call. She had great respect for Bill Stone, who had worked for three years at Rotten Row. He was an extremely caring and able doctor who had the nerve of steel necessary for confinement complications. No matter what time of night or day he was called out, he arrived as if he had stepped out of a "band box". The women used to say, "*Ye would think he's jist stepped oot o' Burton's windae!*"

In the meantime, she had work to do. She checked the babies' heart beats and was reassured that they both were within normal limits. She assisted Maisie to turn in the bed so that she was lying across the bed. She needed this position, as the first twin would need room to hang unobstructed, to bring its head into Maisie's pelvis, ready for delivery. Nell moved the easy chair so that Maisie could put her right foot on it and she moved a chest of drawers over to accommodate the left foot. This served as stirrups like the hospital beds had. Nell did have linen straps that she could have used, but the women felt too confined by them. The straps went over one shoulder and under the opposite arm and supported both legs. Between Maisie's contractions, Nell worked calmly. She wrote out a telephone message requesting the flying squad. She may need this later, as Maisie had a Post Partum Hemorrhage (PPH) with her last baby, which made her high risk for hemorrhaging again, and to further complicate the bleeding possibility, she had been on some anticoagulant therapy for her varicosity! More reasons for Maisie to have a planned hospital confinement!

During each contraction, Nell encouraged Maisie to bear down as much as she could. Maisie knew what was required and her great effort was not in vein. Soon two tiny feet emerged. Another two contractions and the pale body appeared and Nell eased down a loop of the still pulsating umbilical cord (to avoid overstretching the cord as the baby delivered), then she left the baby's body hanging downwards. At the back of her mind she heard her midwifery tutor saying, "*hands off the breech!*"

Although the urge to pull the baby out was tremendous, she knew better. She was waiting for the rest of the baby's body to appear…her adrenaline was running…she was wide awake and aware of every sound and every tiny subtle movement of the baby's body. Down came the shoulders.

"Thank-you God!" Nell prayed.

She knew this meant that the baby's head was free of obstruction, therefore, no locked twins! She heard Shirley open the door, back from the phone box and her father was with her. Hector came in all bright and breezy and the air in the room cooled momentarily, with the cold night air about him. Nell thought that she detected some perfume too—"Evening in Paris," if she was not mistaken. She hoped that Hector was not messing about with another woman.

Hector's face paled as he saw the tiny body hanging there. He could not get near to Maisie, as she lay across the bed and the chair and chest of drawers blocked his way.

He gulped, his eyes fixed on the tiny limp, apparently headless body hanging there and quietly called to her, "I'm here hen, you'll be OK."

Nell asked Hector to stoke the fire up a bit, it was always better to get fathers doing something useful and she did like to encourage their presence at home confinements. She then placed the small piece of old flannelette sheet over the tiny hanging body, as she did not want it to chill. She had warmed the pieces of cloth near the fire for this reason.

Women kept old pieces of sheets and pillowcases for many uses. Well-worn cotton or linen became super soft and made great hankies for children with colds. Paper products were available, but were rough and irritating to the fair Celtic skin. These old pieces of cloth were also used for bandages and bathing skint knees and such like.

At the moment, Nell was using this to keep the tiny body from chilling. Although the kitchen was warm, the difference in temperature from inside Maisie's body to the air temp was great and enough to stimulate the baby to gasp. Nell did not want that to happen, as the baby would inhale vaginal fluids. Nell supported the body and ran her finger along the baby's right arm as she swept the baby's face with it, freeing the right arm.

It was as if her favourite Obstetrician was standing behind her telling her what to do. She had loved his lectures on the whole gamete of midwifery complications during her midwifery training and it had thrilled her, even back then in the classroom. She had also been with him while he delivered the most awkward cases with skill and ease. Yes, she did hear him say, "Now the other arm, just like a cat washing her face." The other arm was free and so Nell once again took her hands off the breech!

She let it hang down and she was waiting for the baby's hairline to appear at the neck. She knew if she acted too soon that she might break the baby's neck. Yes, there was the hairline. She put the Dee-lee aspirator in her mouth (ready to give gentle suction to the baby's nose and mouth) and took the baby's feet in her right hand. Gripping the feet between her fingers, keeping the baby fully extended, she brought the feet up toward the ceiling, making a full arc of 180 degrees. And the face was born. Nell wiped the baby's eyes, using her left hand only and aspirated the mucus from the baby's nose and mouth as the baby gasped and cried. Nell very slowly delivered the rest of the baby's head. Again she heard a voice saying "easy does it, this head had not had time to adjust to the outlet," and then the familiar voice of Dr. Stone saying, "Good job Sister".

Twin one was now born! She noted the time of birth as she laid the baby on a warmed flannelette sheet on Maisie's abdomen and gave him a rub to dry him, then exchanged the sheet quickly for another dry cozy sheet and baby blanket.

Maisie welcomed the child with a, "Hello wee yin! Oh God…look at the hair I think it's rid! Welcome to the world ma wee man!"

Nell cut the cord and covered Maisie and her baby with a warm tartan blanket, made a few brief notes on the labour record and a few words to Dr. Stone. Now for twin two: heartbeat was fine but the position appeared to be transverse; no sign of any action with twin two. Nell examined Maisie to confirm a shoulder presentation. Nell thanked God she had brought Dr. Stone here. He would never take over unless she asked him to do so, but now there was a complication.

After a few brief words with him, Dr. Stone was in action, scrubbing his hands and arms in readiness to turn the baby. He pulled down a leg and Maisie had another breech delivery, this time with a little assistance from the doctor. Bill used a different maneuver to deliver the second baby. The heart rate was falling, so he straddled the baby's body over his upturned, well-scrubbed left arm and slid his middle finger into the baby's mouth. With pointer and ring finger on the chin, while his right hand was placed on the baby's back, the middle finger pushed the baby's head forward and the pointer finger and ring finger pulled on the baby's shoulders.

Another red headed boy, who was a little bit smaller than his big brother of 40 minutes, was born. He appeared to be pale and floppy. Hector McCall's eyes were wide and the expression on his face was one of extreme horror! He thought that the baby was dead! Slowly the baby responded to mouth to mouth breathing and stimulation, and then a piercing cry was heard as everyone in the room laughed out loud in utter relief. The twins were identical.

Maisie coped well with everything and the flying squad did not need to be called after all. She was exhausted as she lay there with her two redheaded babes beside her in bed. Hector McCall matured a little in that hour of his twins' birth. He saw a situation that could have been disastrous, and he was not even aware of the other potential problems that may have befallen Maisie.

Perhaps Hector will give Maisie more help this time round, Nell thought to herself.

So much a part of district midwifery was planning ahead and being ready to take action when necessary. Often the midwife was on her own, with no time to wait for help. Nell did not play with people's lives. She called for help when she thought that she would need it. Her practice was governed by the Scottish Midwives' Board Rules and within that she had her own rules to govern her. There were 206 Scottish Midwives Rules; Nell always thought that there was one for each bone in the body! Sometimes everything worked out well and the help was not necessary, but in Nell's books that was OK. She did not care if she looked like she was being overly cautious. Better to look like that than have a disaster on your hands, with the help you need stuck in a traffic jam 30 minutes away. She knew of too many such cases, some of the stories made the hairs on her neck stand on end. She had a basic love of humanity underlying her caring manner and she definitely did not dice with life.

The dawn was breaking as she prepared to bath the McCall babies in front of the fire. Hector had lifted the ashes and stoked up the fire, so it was really cozy. This was a special time during a home confinement, especially when there were other siblings. It was so different from a hospital delivery where children under twelve were not allowed into visit their mother or new baby except on Saturdays and Sundays between 3 and 4 p.m.

A stupid hospital rule, Nell always thought. There seemed to be too many ex-army ward sisters about in the health service that ruled with a ruthless style of management. They believed that a rule was a rule and should not be broken, irrespective of circumstances! Discretion and common sense were ignored in the face of human need. Nell herself had respect for rules that made sense and a high disrespect for the stupid ones. When she worked in the Maternity wards she often let children in to see their mothers or let the mothers walk out to the day rooms to see the children. It made sense to her that the children needed to know where the mother was, to lessen separation anxiety for all concerned. What difference did the day of the week matter to the infection rate? Children needed to see what was happening. The old Victorian adage, "Children should be seen and not heard," was really old hat now, in the modern sixties.

The other McCall children were up, and a buzz of excitement filled the kitchen. There was Nell with all the McCall siblings gathered round to watch her bathe their new brothers. She knew that there would be questions flying and that her answers would be augmented upon and shared with show and tell at school the next day. Today they all had a holiday, as it was a special day and their sleep had been disturbed. Maisie looked on with restful pride.

The first bath began. There was a popular saying in Glasgow, "You have never been so clean since the midwife bathed you," as they did such a thorough job of it. The bath began by using warm arachis oil. Rex and Lassie moved in to get a good view of the twins and soon there were siblings draped over each of them. The dogs expected this and enjoyed the cuddle from the older children. Often Nell put the baby bath or basin on the floor, but this time Maisie had a new coffee table that she used.

These tables were all the rage at that time. They had a glass covered plywood top and four screw-on legs, which came out at an angle. There was a delicate Japanese sunset scene between the plywood and the glass top—a far cry from the busy dusty Gorbals street scene. Nell made sure that she covered the table well with an old sheet as she had seen many of these tables spoiled by water being spilled and seeping under the glass.

The table's legs soon became wobbly with children using them as a stool. However, for the moment, this one was holding the large white enamel basin that served as the baby bath. Plastic was now in vogue, but this big basin had belonged to Maisie's Granny and had been used to bath Maisie when she was a baby. It was badly chipped round the edge but the main part was white and smooth in contrast to the black rough areas of the chips.

¤

The enameled basin reminded Nell of the ward supplies when she had began her nursing career in the Southern General Hospital. The hospital was in the process of changing from the white enamel to stainless steel "stay-bright" equipment. She remembered snickering when taking down her nursing notes on "how to give a bedpan." Do not give a bedpan with chips in it! Of course she had written in, "without salt and vinegar!" It was just as well that these were personal notes or the Sister Tutor would have had her guts for garters!

¤

Maisie's fire, being the old fire range, had a back water boiler connected to a hot water tank, which was situated just below the ceiling, between the range and the window and below that was a shelved cupboard. From the tank, the hot water pipes ran to the kitchen sink and to the bathroom. There was always plenty of hot water so long as the fire was alight. Glasgow (and Scotland) benefited from the strong engineering heritage of Glasgow University and the strength and quality of the trades.

The range stretched across about five feet, the fire was situated about the center of it and on the right there was the gas hob and two ovens: one heated by gas and the other by the coal fire. Above the industrious range towered the mantle piece, which was a domain unto itself.

The mantle clock with a loud tick and often a chiming mechanism (traditional wedding present from the Best Man at the wedding) had pride of place in the center. Two matching white gilded "wally" dugs (dogs), were placed one at each end of the mantelpiece, looking at each other with that knowing look, as if they had witnessed everything before! If the "wally" dugs were not there, then there would be two sitting Alsatian dogs or two cherub looking girls, either holding out their skirts in a curtsy or holding a bunch of cherries.

Between the dogs and the clock were items that were deemed dangerous to children, such as matches, the mothers purse and the sweetie jar.

The ornaments were termed "wally" meaning that they were made of clay. Some of them had been well fired while some of the cheaper ones that had not been fired broke easily. When this happened, the children could play with the chalk shards. Nell always knew when there had been the demise of a "wally" dog as one could play hopscotch on the pavement for miles! These large ornaments were going out of fashion since the new houses did not have a kitchen range. The cooking was done in a kitchenette and the coal fire (with back boiler to heat the water) was in a tiled fireplace in the living room. The mantelpieces were respectively smaller and of course did not hold so much.

The warmed arachis oil anointed the small flat-topped head of the first McCall twin, on down over the shoulders, out to the arms, over the body, back and front and down the legs in one continuous motion of Nell's hands. She loved the feel of the oil on the baby's skin and she was able to assess the muscle tone of the baby while performing this task. Nell wrapped the baby up again in the towel, leaving only the head uncovered. Then, she bathed the eyes with soft cotton wool balls, one for each eye, and shampooed the fiery red curls and combed through the hair to ensure that all the blood was gone.

When Nell placed the baby in the bath, the children chorused an "Awh he's dead wee Sister."

Two of the boys were sniggering and eventually the older one said, "His wullie's awefie wee Sister."

They were all giggling now and nudging one another, but they were astute and had noticed that this twin had undescended testicles and the little scrotum was small and ridged and did not have the usual slack skin of the scrotum.

"Don't you worry, he is small now but when he grows everything else will grow too," Nell assured them.

The cord always fascinated them and that took their attention next. There were "Oohs and Ahhs" and "Ughs" about the cord.

One great benefit of the old tenement kitchen was that everything happened there; Maisie was in bed in the recess, with the curtains pulled open. From this vantage position she could oversee almost everything that was going on in the room. She could see the fire in the range where the cooking was done, the sink in front of the window and the kitchen table in the middle of the room, which was the hub of family life. If only the kitchen table could talk, what tales it would tell!

Now here she was, four days later, sitting at the kitchen table talking to Nell about the twins feeding. Maisie was looking tired but she said that she had had eight hours of sleep, broken in the middle of course. Hector had helped her feed the twins at three a.m. He was now making up his lost sleep in the other room. He fed one by bottle as she breastfed the other. Maisie said she was going to do that alternately so that the twins would each get some breast milk. It was wonderful how sensible and down to earth Maisie was. Nell always encouraged the women to work things out for themselves and only offered suggestions along the way.

"Hector's eldest sister, Ina's comin' tae see us the day…and she'll wait till aboot eight the night. She'll be a good help. I like Ina best of all and the kids just love her. Shirley's baked Ina a cake and said she'd hide it incase Brian and Archie got their paws on it. She's a great girl, is ma Shirley an' she's been a great help with the feedin." Maisie was rattling on ten to the dozen and Nell was pleased that she was having help today.

"Try to get a couple of hours rest when Ina comes in," Nell suggested. "That will help your milk supply too. I've counted up what each twin has had since last night and they are doing far better now. I was a bit worried, but I'll weigh them today and then again at the end of the week. You will see their wee cheeks begin to fill out when they start to put weight on."

"Right Sister, an Ah'll keep a note of how much they take like Ah did before…an' oh Ah nearly forgoat. Look at whit ma Shirley made…she made up a chart fur each twin."

Maisie proudly presented Nell with the two charts. They had been made out of pages from a scrapbook and the twins' names were printed on each: Douggie McCall, and Danny McCall. Shirley had ruled out two columns. At the top of the first column was printed "time he fed at" and at the top of the second column was "how much he took."

"These are wonderful Maisie. You will have to keep these as a keepsake when you are finished with them."

"I never thought of that Sister…but ah wull dae jist that too."

Nell completed the postnatal visit and bathed the babies for Maisie. This was a good way to examine the babies, who were active and warm and had good colour. Bathing the babies also gave Maisie time to talk, and from what she said and how she said it, Nell was able to assess how she was coping. All was well with the McCall twins and their mammy. Nell buttoned her double breasted coat, slipped the belt through the green bakelite buckle, tugged to tighten it, lifted her case, and was on her way.

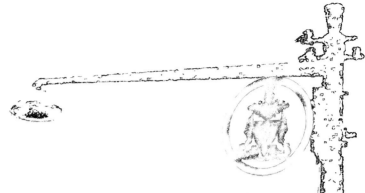

Chapter 4
Isa Carmichael

The sleet battered against Nell's back as she trudged along Eglinton Street. She glanced in Ian Fair's car showroom window as she passed by and imagined what it would be like to drive that beautiful, shiny black, highly polished Rover 100, complete with the red leather upholstery and gleaming oak finished dashboard. Nell loved to daydream. Ever since she was a small girl she could become lost in a daydream. It got her into trouble many times.

¤

Once, when she was about ten years old, she was sitting at her school desk staring out through the classroom window at the Glasgow Corporation electricians while they serviced the street lamp. There was a lorry that had a hydraulic hoist to take the man up to the height of the lamp post and another two men to see that he did it right and to hand him the new light bulbs. Nell was so engrossed in what they were doing, and imagined herself up in the hoist, that she had tuned out on the history lesson in progress.

Mr. Tain, the teacher, who saw Nell staring out of the window asked, "Nell, what was King Arthur doing while the cakes were burning?"

The girl next to her gave her an almighty dig in the ribs with her elbow, which abruptly brought Nell into the present and she blurted out, "Changing the light bulbs, Sir!"

Everybody laughed! Immediately Nell blushed to the roots of her hair.

"Big riddy, big riddy," a couple of the boys chanted as the laugh-

ter was subsiding. "Big riddy" was referring to her blushing, which she failed to have any control over. She hated it.

¤

Yes! A big luxurious Rover and a chauffeur of course, to swan about the Gorbals in—that would set the tongues a chattering, eh! How about that hen? she asked herself.

There was a new patient, Isa Carmichael, whom Nell was anxious to see; so, instead of going home for lunch after her morning visits were done, she headed for the Easy Eats Café. Isa Carmichael had just moved to the area and her expected date of delivery was in two weeks and, as Nell didn't know anything about her, she wanted to meet her as soon as possible. Midwives needed to know the entire patient's past history before the onset of labour so that there would be fewer nasty surprises!

She pushed open the door of the Easy Eats Café and was greeted by, "Oh Sister, your drookit, gees a hoddy your coat an Ah'll hing it beside the hoat water boiler tae dry aff," said Geoff McCarty, the proprietor.

"Thanks Geoff. I didn't even get time to get the nylon rain coat out of my bag before that last downpour hit me!"

"How's it goin Sister? Here sit here near the heater an Ah'll get your tea right away hen, jist the way ye like it; not too strong wi' a wee doad o' lemon," bustled May McCarty, Geoff's wife.

"That's whit ye call a Russian Tea," smiled Geoff.

"Well, the sister's aye rushin' anyway," grinned May as she squeezed passed him.

"I'll just phone the office to see if there are any messages for me—won't be a jiffy," Nell informed Geoff, as she headed for the public phone just inside the café doorway.

There was nothing quite like the taste of Ayrshire bacon with a fried egg in a Scottish morning roll and a steaming hot cup of tea, thought Nell. It sure did warm the cockles of your heart on a raw winter's day like today. She loved the taste of the bacon fat, and as a child she had been encouraged to eat all the fat on meat to keep out the cold and to put a "skin on your keech." She always thought the latter expression was a bit disgusting, but she ate the fat just the same!

Nell had known Geoff and May before they took over the Easy Eats Café. She had delivered their last baby, James, about three years ago. Geoff was a big man, six feet in his stocking soles, with a good physique, which he kept trim by being as active as he could be. Prior to the accident, he had played football but now he only managed to coach the junior team. Geoff had balding dirty fair hair, sky blue eyes and a neat mustache.

In days gone by Geoff had worked as a welder in Fairfield's shipyard on Govan Road. There had been a severe accident there just over two years ago when external scaffolding collapsed. Two men died and three were badly injured. Geoff was one of the injured and had sustained a fractured pelvis and femur. He had spent many months in the orthopedic ward at the Southern General Hospital.

Geoff knew that he could never return to work as a welder, so he decided to open the Easy Eats Café with the compensation payout. He had a stint at being a cook in the Royal Navy in his younger days so he had some training. He would miss the camaraderie of his shipmates, but he knew he was lucky to be alive, so he wasn't going to tempt fate any more. This way he could pace himself with the chronic back pain. He sure did keep the café "ship shape and Bristol fashion."

Nell liked to give them the business when she was in the area. If Nell had a Student Midwife allocated to her, she would arrange to meet her here, at the Café. It was easy to get to and from Hospital Nurses' homes, as it was on the main bus route. Nell knew that she could always contact them by phone at the café if there was a sudden change of plan. It was good too, that they had a public phone inside the doorway to the café as she often sent children to them with a message to relay to a doctor. Nell always squared up the cash with Geoff as soon as she saw him again. Geoff would write any message from the doctor for Nell, put it in an envelope, give it to the wee messenger and usually give them a Tunnock's caramel wafer as a treat as he told them to hurry back to the Sister. Geoff was a kind man—the salt of the earth. Nell appreciated this help so much and only used it if she was in real need.

There was a cozy big room at the back of the restaurant, just off the kitchen, where May's mother, Sadie, looked after wee Jim all day, as well as the other two children, when they came home from school. Sadie was a good soul. Nell first met her at a confinement of one of Sadie's neighbours. She was small in stature and motherly rotund.

Nell remembered her joking, "Guid gear goes into small bulk," when someone said that she was the height of nonsense! She was always smiling and had endless energy. Sadie was at her neighbour's confinement holding the fort and seeing to the needs of the family.

It was great the way that the women stuck by each other when a baby was on the way or if there was a family crisis. Some of the men, too, would lend a hand, as long as whatever they did looked macho-like. May had peace of mind with her mother looking after wee Jim close at hand; after all they nearly did not have him at all.

"Who could I trust more than ma mammy?" May had once asked Nell. "You cannae whack a mother's love, Sister."

Nell nodded her head in agreement and thought of her own mother, who died when she was a child. "Yes! And when it's gone there's no getting it back. And nothing can fully replace it either, only a huge ache fills the gap."

When Geoff was in hospital following his injuries, May hired a baby-sitter for her three kids while she went to visit him. The baby sitter was a girl of eighteen and May had known her for about six months. Kristy had been baby-sitting for May a few times and all seemed to go well. However, one Sunday afternoon things went all wrong. A couple of teenage boys appeared at the door with some beer. Kristy let them in and they settled down to watch the match (semi-final football match for the Scottish cup) on television. At that time, not many people had television and Kristy told her boyfriend to come and visit—May knew about that.

May's children, Roger, eight and Crystal, five, along with the eleven month old baby, Jim, been watching a children's special program at the time. They had to go and find something else to do. A few minutes later another five teenagers arrived. This was not what Kristy had wanted. She only invited her boyfriend, who had arrived with his brother in tow just shortly before.

Kristy opened the door of the ground floor flat and asked them to leave, but a row broke out! There was a bit of pushing and shoving. Soon there was shouting and then some fisticuffs were flying. Suddenly there was a horrifying screech of brakes from the road outside and as the din fell, they could hear Crystal howling and sobbing. Kristy paled and gulped as her heart leapt into her mouth. She flew out of the close to find wee Jim crawling on the road inches away from the front of a gigantic lorry with Crystal, blinded by tears, trying to pick him up!

"If Ah hundae seen the wee lassie running out o' the close mooth Ah wudnae hae seen the wean!" the agitated, but relieved, lorry driver hastily explained to the quickly growing crowd.

"Ah thought she was chasing a dug."

Kristy, shaking with emotion, gathered Jim up in her arms. "C'mon

Crystal let's get back inside hen. Thank God you saw him crawling out among all that stramash."

The troublesome youths had disappeared "like snow aff a dyke!"

The impact of what almost happened had a profound effect. Kristy never baby-sat again for anyone nor did May ever hire any baby-sitter again. If her mother or sister could not look after the children, she took them with her or didn't go out.

"Another wee cup o' tea Sister?" May's inquiring voice brought Nell out of her dream.

"Yes thanks May," Nell replied. "It's a good cuppa."

"…an' will ye huv a wee biscuit or a cream bun to keep your second cup company?" May offered as she poured out the steaming tea into Nell's cup.

May was a wee bit taller and slimmer than her mother was but just as cheery and bouncy. She brought out the best in people with her upbeat ways and sparkling hazel coloured eyes. Her hair, a force to be reckoned with, was mousy brown, strongly permed and defied all gravity.

"Oh! I think that it is a cream bun kind of a day," said Nell smiling. "I shouldn't but I will. Thanks for twisting my arm, May."

They both smiled with a nod and a wink. May brought the cream bun on a china tea plate. The pattern was one of Nell's favorites—the Tree of India pattern. Nell had a tea set in this pattern at home.

"Thanks May, I will enjoy this," she tapped the loose icing sugar off the bun in readiness to sinking her teeth into the freshly whipped cream and soft tea-bread. She usually was left with an icing sugar mustache! Such was life!

Warmed and fortified, Nell got her dry, heated coat from Geoff who helped her on with the weighty garment.

"It feels like an electric blanket Geoff. Thanks, that's grand. I'll put on the nylon raincoat on top before I go out."

Nell paid the bill, buttoned up her green double breasted coat, which was warm all over, slid the green belt through the green bakelite buckle and pulled to tighten it. Then she donned the green nylon raincoat, lifted her case, and headed into the inclement weather once more.

Nell strode at a good pace toward Abbotsford Place where Isa Carmichael lived. She found the number that she was looking for and turned into the close and trudged up the spiral staircase to the B side. She found "Carmichael" on a piece of paper stuck to the wall at the side of the door of one top floor flats. The door opened as soon as she rang the bell. A large cheery faced woman appeared. She wore a blue and white frilled pinny on over a thick red jumper and a red Robertson tartan maternity pinafore. She had thick support stockings on and her feet bulged out of a pair of gent's brown checked slippers. This was Isa Carmichael in person!

"Come away in Sister, I'm pleased to see you. I was expecting you but what a cold driech day it is," said Isa in a warm welcoming way.

She had a soft Ayrshire accent and had lived most of her days in the sea side town of Troon which lies to the south west of Glasgow. Isa had rented two of the rooms in this spacious, six-apartment flat, and had shared use of the kitchen and bathroom. She showed Nell into the larger of the rooms where a coal fire crackled in the grate. There was a big fireguard round the whole hearth to keep the toddler at bay. Nell thought that these guards were better than the small spark guards that closely covered the grate. The larger guard was so useful to dry or heat up clothes and was strong if a child fell against it.

In one corner of the room sat a double bed that was covered with a down quilt and matching bed spread in pale pink satin. Beside the bed was a child's cot that was neatly made up with a good quality blue and pink checked cot blanket, which had its ends well tucked in round the mattress. Some soft toys were neatly lined up along the bottom of the cot and a well-worn one-eyed teddy was propped up at the top end.

This was the largest room in the flat and was the original sitting room. It accommodated a velour covered three piece suite, a large kitchen table with six chairs, a kitchen cabinet, and a Welsh dresser complete with a display of willow patterned plates. The three-seater couch was placed directly in front of the fire with the large armed matching lounge chairs on either side of the Cumberland stone fireplace. The fireplace was decorated with a vine and grape design across the top, just under the mantle piece. On its left side was a brass coal scuttle and inside the fireguard at the right, stood a tall standing brass companion set consisting of tongs, shovel, poker and brush. Each piece had a large thistle on the top. The brush was characteristically placed the farthest from the fire. There was a Westminster clock in the center of the mantelpiece, which chimed the quarter hour when Nell walked in. This was comfortable showing no apparent poverty. Nell wondered why Isa was in two sublet rooms. No doubt she would hear the story of Isa Carmichael from Isa herself in due course.

Nell sat down to take Isa's medical and maternity history and to give Isa a full prenatal visit. She found out that this was Isa's fourth pregnancy.

She had 16-year-old twins, Sarah and Tom and a girl, Emma, who was 13. These two pregnancies were by Isa's first husband, Donald Robertson, a lawyer in Troon. Donald died eight years ago of a very rapid bone cancer. She remarried five years ago to Jake Carmichael, who had been at school with Isa and Donald. He was a lawyer too and things worked out well. Elizabeth was born two years ago and the new baby expected soon.

Six months ago her world was turned upside down when Jake was sentenced to three years imprisonment for embezzlement. He was incarcerated in Barlinney Prison, in Glasgow. Jake had been involved in a big business deal that went wrong and he appeared to be the fall guy. They lost their house and most of their savings. Isa had been promised a house, in Cardonald, which at the last minute, fell through, and this was the best that the she could find at such short notice. Isa came to Glasgow to be nearer Jake.

"He is a soft big soul Sister," shared Isa, "and has just been taken to the cleaners. I really don't think he has a crooked bone in his body. He was just out of his depth with those business sharks! We will be fine if he can hack the prison life. He has set the ball rolling for an appeal, but these things take time."

"Yes, they do take time," said Nell empathizing.

"Financially, I'm OK as the government looks after me to a point, and the kids have their schooling paid for by their Grandpa Robertson. Tom is at Glasgow Academy and the girls are at Laurel Bank School. I feel bad for them living here. They try to hide their school uniforms from the kids here and of course they don't want to bring any friends home to these rooms. I am optimistic that I will get one of those "Meikle and MacTaggart" houses in Cardonald after Christmas, and that would be great as my sister Irene lives there. I have requested a five room apartment and have a few contacts pulling for me."

"That would be good to be near your sister," said Nell.

This all came pouring out of Isa like water from a dam when the floodgates have just been opened.

She went on, "In the meantime I am trying to make the most of this and I have the baby to look forward to."

Nell took Isa's blood pressure, which was elevated a bit. Isa had a copy of her prenatal records from the midwife in Troon to give to Nell. This was so essential and Nell noticed that Isa's BP had been highish most of the pregnancy. Nell went through the house to the bathroom to test Isa's urine sample. She visibly shivered as she crossed the large unheated hallway to the bathroom, which was equally as cold. She looked up at the electric heater and saw that it was controlled by a "shilling-in-the-slot-meter". The heater hadn't a hope in hell of heating the vast space, unless it burned for at least half an hour. It was the same for the hot water electric emersion heater. Nell noted that it was a costly affair to have a bath in the dead of winter in sub-let rooms. Why were living essentials so costly in Scotland?

¤

Many people in these situations took a bath in the public bathhouses, which were usually attached to the public swimming pools and the public laundry facility or wash houses, lovingly called the "Steamie". The individual baths were housed in single rooms and were quite private. The whole complex was at least warm, with a steamy sort of heat.

¤

Nell didn't linger when testing Isa's urine. Just as she thought—strongly positive for protein. She had noticed Isa's swollen ankles on the way in and would now check for any other signs of swelling. Swollen ankles on their own were to be expected with every pregnancy, where as swelling anywhere else was indicative of "pre-eclampsia", and Isa would have to go into hospital if that was so.

Nell completed her exam to discover that there did not seem to be any other swelling. Nell also planned to phone the Doc and get a urine sample sent to the lab to find out if there was another reason for the proteinuria. Isa did want to have a home confinement, for the obvious reasons. Her sister would come and stay for a week; she had arranged a week's holiday from her work from the time Isa went into labour. Nell would discuss this case with Dr. Martin. Often women with essential high blood pressure succumb to a superimposed pre-eclampsia.

She felt that at the moment Isa was OK to stay at home. It seemed that her blood pressure has always been on the high side, so it might not be the pregnancy that has elevated it.

"Will you take a cup of tea, Sister?" asked Isa when the exam was over.

"Yes thanks," said Nell "but you must let me make it."

When patients asked this at regular visits, it meant that they wanted to talk more. Isa had an old kettle simmering away on the fire, which meant that she did not have to go across the frozen hallway to the communal kitchen. The actual grate had two round iron plates six inches in diameter, which could swivel towards or away from the fire. A kettle or pot was quite steady sitting on them and was a great saver on fuel and time. Nell lifted the kettle, which was half covered in coal soot, off the fire, using an oven glove, made the tea and handed Isa a cup.

They spoke about what Isa would need for the confinement, as Glasgow Corporation did things a bit differently from the Ayrshire District. She needed to look out an ashet, or a large soup plate as a receptacle for the placenta. The two women talked over many things concerning the impending delivery, the children and the prison visiting. Isa was keeping up a strong front and making a comfortable home for the children. It was not easy for them to be living this double standard; posh paying school each day, then home to low cost sub-let housing conditions. Tom had school rugby on a Saturday. His Uncle Bill picked him and his younger cousin up from the rugby and he stayed overnight with Bill's family. His Aunt laundered his rugby gear ready for school practice and then they dropped him off at Air Cadets on Sunday afternoon.

Isa said, "I miss him at the weekend, but I feel he needs some male company, so when Bill offered and he wanted to go, I agreed. Tom has a lot of school homework during the week, as there is fierce competition and high standards to contend with."

The second room that Isa had was a large bedroom in which Tom and the girls slept. They had always been used to rooms of their own and now they had to share. Isa had divided the room using two wardrobes and two dressing tables as a room divider. Sarah's dressing table backed on to the back of Tom's wardrobe and Tom's dresser backed on to the back of a large double wardrobe, which the girls shared. Isa was pleased that she still had all her furniture, some of which was stored in her father-in-law's basement. The room still had space for three single beds, with bedside cabinets and a couple of big chairs at the fireplace. There was a table at the window and a trunk full of toys. Isa put Elizabeth down for a sleep and showed the room to Nell.

"It is like a campsite, but I wanted them to have their own space. I have given them as much of their own stuff as possible, so they don't feel totally and utterly lost," Isa explained.

"There is enough room here for the three of them. I think that you have done a great job," said Nell, looking round.

"It is cold in here," said Isa, rubbing the tops of her arms with the palms of her hands. "I bring a kindling through from the other fire about four o'clock to set this one going for the evening. Tom and Sarah study in here, since there is too much noise in the other room. I do have electric heaters, but I can't keep up with the coin meter."

Nell nodded knowingly. Some landlords made money from this arrangement and never shared the coin rebate with the tenants.

The two women returned to the other room where little Elizabeth had fallen fast asleep in the cot. Isa showed Nell the woven Moses' basket for the baby that was hidden behind the cot.

"This has been in the family for years. I repainted it for Elizabeth. That's a new quilt and bumper pads that I made for this little one," she said as she patted her belly.

"Isa you are all set for this baby and I think you are a real brick coping with all you are coping with," said Nell.

Isa sat down and burst into tears, "I'm sorry Sister. I'll be OK in a wee minute but sometimes I think I can't go on. It is so good to talk to you, but I miss my friends and family in Troon. My sister in Cardonald will be over to see me at the weekend. I really have a lot to be thankful for."

"Just you let it out and have a good bubble to yourself. Don't bottle things up. You have every right to feel as you do," reassured Nell.

The two women continued to talk about the approaching labour and Nell gave Isa a list of phone numbers. Isa appeared to be calmer.

"I'll pop in to see you on Monday to check your blood pressure and maybe we will have the result of the urine test if you see the doctor tomorrow."

"Thanks Sister, I feel better now that I have met you."

"Every time Elizabeth goes for a sleep please lie down yourself, Isa, you really need as much rest as you can get," implored Nell as she put her coats on.

"Yes Sister I'll do that, I do feel a wee bit wabbit just now."

"Right then Isa you do that and I'll see myself out," Nell said quietly, not to waken Elizabeth in the cot. "Cheerio then, see you on Monday," whispered Nell and with that she buttoned her double breasted coat, slipped the green belt through the green bakelite buckle, tugged to tighten it, lifted her case, and left through the Siberian-like hallway.

When Monday came; it was cold but dry. Nell knocked on Isa's door. Perhaps there is no one in? Nell knocked again. The door opened and a tired looking Isa, in her dressing gown, opened the door.

"Come away in Sister, sorry I'm a bit slow today," said Isa softly.

"How are you doing?" inquired Nell as she followed Isa into the big room.

In the bright day light Nell could see that Isa was far from well. She was "peely wally" and tired looking and Nell could see that her face was puffy with dark rings round her eyes.

"Sister I have this pain in my middle between my ribs just here," Isa pointed high between her ribs.

Nell took Isa's blood pressure, which was elevated from her previous reading. Nell found protein plus, plus in Isa's specimen. The urinalysis done by the laboratory had discounted infection. Nell looked at Isa's hands and her fingers were puffy.

"I had a struggle to get my rings off," said Isa.

Nell listened in to the baby through the Pinnards stethoscope and was relieved to hear the reassuring gallop of the baby's heartbeat.

"The baby's heart beat is fine in there," said Nell smiling to Isa.

"That's a blessing," said Isa, stroking Elizabeth's head.

Isa has pre-eclampsia which is rapidly fulminating into eclampsia, thought Nell.

"Isa you will have to go into Rotten Row. It is not safe for you or the baby to continue like this. I am sure that they will induce you today." Nell was looking Isa straight in the eye.

"I really feel awful Sister. Whatever you think is best, I'll do," conceded Isa.

"A few phone calls and we will have everything organized; the doctor, the ambulance, the almoner, your sister, and Tom's uncle. That's all I need," said Nell.

"Now Isa, please just lie in bed till the ambulance comes. I won't leave Elizabeth till the Almoner gets here. Don't worry now, this time next week you will be back home."

Nell gathered up the numbers she needed and the key to get back in and left Isa in bed with Elizabeth, who was colouring in a book. Nell headed for the Easy Eats Café.

"Good morning Geoff," greeted Nell. "I have a bit of an emergency this morning and I need to use the phone.

"Come away through to the back and use our private phone, there's less din in there Sister," urged Geoff.

"Well if you are sure, that would be just the ticket, thanks Geoff," said Nell heading for the back room.

She knew there was no time to lose. When she had finished her phone calls she headed back to Isa's and packed a small case for her and a larger case for Elizabeth. Isa told Nell where everything was. Nell was amazed at how organized Isa was. Irene, Isa's sister, would see to the others.

The Almoner arrived before the ambulance. Elizabeth had met the Almoner before and didn't protest going with her. Nell was pleased that Elizabeth didn't make a fuss, as Isa's blood pressure was really high. It was as though she knew that things were tense.

Isa gave Elizabeth a kiss. "See you soon with Aunt Irene," she smiled at her, knowing it would only be for a few hours till Isa's sister got home from work. Nell sat in the ambulance with Isa as it sped away with the siren whining.

The day passed quickly for Nell, as she was busy with pre- and post-natal visits. Whenever she was not actively thinking about something, Isa Carmichael and her plight would float back into her conscious mind.

"Glasgow Royal Maternity, yes I'll put you through to the labour ward," the hospital operator's voice replied.

"A boy at five minutes past six, both well." Nell knew Senga, the hospital Sister there, so she asked after Isa's condition.

"Just as well you got her in as soon as you did Nell, as she was beginning to twitch when we got her to the labour ward," Senga said.

"Yes! An eclamptic fit at home is not desirable. Thank goodness for a good ambulance service. The ambulance men were superb," replied Nell. "How is the baby? How small is he?"

"Yes, five pounds two, just a wee scrag of a thing, but by God he has a good pair of lungs. I think he'll be a piper for sure!"

"Thanks Senga, Isa was an essential hypertension with a superimposed pre-eclampsia. I thought that the baby would be a wee thing. Can you tell Isa I called, and I will come into see her on Thursday when I'm up at the office."

"Sure I will Nell, ta ta the noo."

Nell put the receiver down. There was a smile on her face as she thought, thank God they are both through the worse. There was still a risk of Isa having an Eclamptic fit but she would be sedated and under observation.

Nell had done a special study of pre-eclampsia for a project during her midwifery training; the subject fascinated her.

It was the Greeks who gave the name "eclampsia" to women who had convulsions in pregnancy. The word means "sudden flash out." It wasn't until later that the term pre-eclampsia was used, when it was noted that women with high blood pressure, protein in their urine and generalized puffy-ness were more likely to have eclamptic fits. It was noted on postmortem that the brain, the kidneys and the liver were all affected. The pain Isa had was over her liver.

Nell thought of wee baby Carmichael blowing the bagpipes! Senga knew how to diffuse a situation! A great nurse and midwife was Senga, and a nice happy, bubbly person. Nell had trained with her and they had had many an escapade in their younger days. They used to tease her about her name. She came from three generations of Agnes' and her mother wanted a change without upsetting her granny and great-granny. The nurses would tease her with, "Here comes backward Agnes!" She would just laugh or turn and walk backwards.

"Hello Sister," said Isa cheerily, "let me introduce you to Master David Carmichael."

There he was just after a breastfeed, full to the gunnels. His lips were pouting, showing off a few sucking blisters. His eyes were closed in slumber with the occasional flicker. His face and baldhead were flushed by the bosom warmth, and arms and legs sprawled over the flannelette wrap, which had pink and blue bunnies at play. He was a tiny wee mite, just a handful.

"Well then, hello wee man!" said Nell softly, as she took his little hand on her fore finger and stroked his fingers with her thumb. "We'll need to get you a piano, you have long slender fingers, cherub."

"We have one in storage," said Isa, smiling.

"Is there any arrangement for Jake to visit?" asked Nell.

"The hospital Almoner had been in contact with the prison and Jake is scheduled to see us tomorrow. I am really looking forward to seeing him. I'm glad he is coming to the hospital, as it would upset him more if he saw where we are living. He has enough to cope with getting through each day."

"Isa I know the visit will go well. They have a visitor's room here and you will have a nice private visit." Nell thought of Isa worrying about Jake's lot and not the lot that has fallen on her own shoulders.

"I'll come and see you when you get home Isa, Oh! Here is a wee gift, I nearly forgot." Nell reached in her bag for a card and small parcel.

"Thanks Sister, I'll open it now," Isa said as she untied the blue ribbon to reveal two hand knitted baby's helmets, one in blue and one in white three-ply Paton's Beehive baby wool.

"Those will fit him perfectly Sister, thanks very much."

"Well when I heard his weight and I knew that you didn't have any tiny hats I thought it would be a good idea. They'll be snug and that's what's needed in this weather."

"Can't wait to get him home," said a tired Isa.

"It won't be too long now and you do need a rest," Nell reassured her.

"Cheerio Sister, and thanks again."

"Isa it was you that did all the work and the hats were my pleasure. See you when you get home. Just relax now." Nell gave Isa a wave as she left the ward.

She left Rotten Row and headed down Montrose Street's steep hill towards the City Chambers and George Square. The Glasgow City Chambers is an impressive building that held dear memories for Nell. She was glad to be a Glaswegian, and was proud of this landmark facing out on to George Square, with its flower beds, park benches, towering historical statues and, last but by no means least, the grey lion adorned cenotaph in front of the City Chambers. The City Chambers itself housed beautiful surprises, including Italian marble staircases, oak paneled chambers and the grand Banquet hall with sky high murals. Nell's first time in the City Chambers was a school tour. She had often been in the Banquet Hall for various functions including the annual Christmas card sale, during which charities could have a stall to sell cards to the public.

George Square was as busy as usual, with people meeting there or crossing over as a short cut to Queens Street. Nell headed for Renfield Street and the bus home. As she was boarding the bus, two boys came clambering down the stairs and nearly crashed into her.

"Watch that green wuman. Don't knoak her doon," said the follower, as the leader swung on the rail and jumped off the bus.

A couple of live wires. Not a care in the world. Long may that be true for them, Nell thought as she glanced after them, as they jostled each other along the pavement, giggling as they went. She loved to see happy children. She wished in her heart happiness for the Carmichael children and their parents.

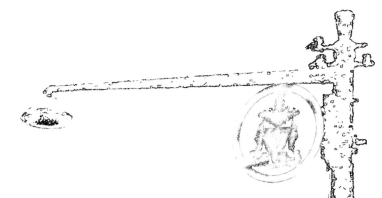

Chapter 5
Hazel Brown

Nell phoned the central office on Ingram St. from the Easy Eats Café at lunchtime.

"It's Sister Dickson here, are there any messages for me, Miss MacGreggor?" Nell knew that she had three patients near or at their confinement dates.

"Yes Sister Dickson, a Mrs. Brown, on Portugal Street is in labour. Someone phoned at 10:30 a.m. saying that her contractions were every five minutes. We have sent a Student Midwife out with the Gas and Air machine," reported the superintendent.

"Oh! Thanks Miss MacGreggor. I will run over there right away. I'm only a few streets away."

"Now Sister dinna fash yersel' for as sure as God's in Govan, the Student will cope fine till you get there. She has a delivery case with her and she is a bright lassie with plenty common sense."

"Oh! I'm just minutes away, thanks Miss MacGreggor, I'll phone you later, or get a message to you before five o'clock."

"Good Sister, now you take your time, there are plenty of prizes you know."

Nell liked Lucy MacGreggor. She was the salt of the earth, never panicked, always had a Glasgow expression for everything, which in itself put things in perspective, and she looked for the best in everyone. She had been a Domiciliary Midwife in Govan in her younger years and worked there all through the blitz. She had some stories to tell of wartime midwifery. She told Nell that when the air raid sirens went off, some women would go into premature labour and many babies were lost.

One positive thing about the administrative staff, Nell thought, was that they really knew what the midwives had to deal with, day in and day out. Unlike one particular Hospital Administrator, who was a regular attendee at the Royal College of Midwives meetings and delighted in running down the district midwives because they did some grocery shopping in their uniforms on the way home from visits. Had the woman any sense at all? What were they supposed to do on a 24 hour on call schedule? The District midwives ignored her acidic comments at these meetings as the old adage held true in this scenario: where ignorance is bliss it is folly to be wise.

Nell was not bothered, but this negativity did seep under her skin at times. The caliber of some of these promoted hospital midwives left a lot to be desired. The perception of power does strange things to some people.

Nell gathered up her stuff and said to Geoff, "I'm off to a confinement so I may use the phone later."

"Huv ye no time for a wee quick cuppa' afore ye run?"

"Wish I had the time, Geoff, but I'll need to scoot today," Nell replied.

"OK Sister, cheerio the noo…"

"I may see you later," and with that Nell's green coat swirled out of the Café door.

It didn't take Nell long to reach the Brown's place. This was one girl, Hazel Brown, who Nell felt needed a good shake. This would be her fourth baby in four years; nothing wrong with that on its own, but the kids were neglected and the house was far from clean. The children looked like wee poor waifs of things with dirty faces, the customary dreep from the nose, dirty clothes that were usually unseasonable and hair that was unbrushed and matted. Nell felt there was no need for this, as Hazel had been well looked after as a child. Her husband, Bernie, had a regular job as a printer, so there was steady money coming into the house.

Hazel puzzled Nell. Nell knew that her highland grandmother and grandfather on Elizabeth Street in Ibrox had brought her up. Her grandmother, Bell, was from Lewis and had come to Glasgow to train as a nurse at the Victoria Infirmary. She met Hazel's grandfather, Hugh, who was from Islay. Hugh was in the Merchant Navy then and later worked as a long-distance lorry driver. Bell and Hugh had one daughter, Lizzie.

Hazel was born out of wedlock when Lizzie was eighteen. This shook

Bell and Hugh but they both fell in love with the new baby Hazel. Soon after Hazel's birth, Lizzie went to work in London as a receptionist in a posh hotel. Bell and Hugh brought Hazel up with little help from Lizzie. Hazel would go for a two week holiday down to London to see her mother in the summer time and Lizzy would come up to Glasgow in December for a week. Hazel's grandparents did everything for her. She was well educated and worked as a shorthand typist in a local school before she got married. She was a beautiful bride, as the wedding picture on the wall displayed. Nell wondered if Hazel had a deep resentment for not sharing more of her mother's life.

Hazel did not seem to have a clue about housework. Bernie's parents had given them a wedding present of a beautiful lounge suite and a fitted carpet, which, at that time, was the very latest in fashion. Nell went in one day and found her trying to sweep the new fitted carpet with a dry mop! And two of the children were sitting on the couch eating a "piece on jam" and the jam was dripping on to the velvety fabric of the couch. She let the children run around without nappies and they would urinate on the floor or the chairs, but it did not seem to bother Hazel. The smell lingered and the guff hit you as soon as the door was opened. That unclean, heavy smell was so distinctive!

Hazel always kept her babies nice, but when they began to crawl she became almost disinterested in them. Nell had noticed this trend with other women and their children. Mind you, Hazel usually fell pregnant about that time, so that might have had something to do with it.

When her grandparents came to visit, old Bell would spend her time cleaning and cooking while Hugh, the good old soul, would gather up the dirty clothes, put them in the pram and take them to the launderette. Unfortunately, Hazel would just let things slip till they visited again. She did not see her mother often. What made her tick to a different rhythm from her grandparents did puzzle Nell. Was it laziness, pure and simple? Or was it a case of "act daft and get a free hurl"? Bernie came in from work and would start to do the housework, then her grandparents would do the major clean ups—Hazel ambled on regardless. Did Hazel suffer from depression?

Dear knows what the Student will think of the Hazel Brown situation, Nell thought to herself as she knocked on the Brown's pillar–box, red painted door. A visibly relieved Student Midwife opened it.

"Oh! Sister I'm glad to see you, I'm Student Midwife Blair," said Chris

Blair hurriedly, as she grasped her watch in one hand and the door handle in the other.

"Hello Nurse Blair, how's Hazel doing?" inquired Nell.

"Her contractions are coming every three minutes lasting 50 – 60 seconds and have increased in strength since I arrived at 11:15. I would say they are strong now. She has heavy show but her membranes are intact I think, because I can't detect any fluid. The foetal heart rate is 120 to 132 beats per minute between contractions."

Nurse Blair took a few big breaths as she looked at Nell, who smiled and nodded in reassurance for her to continue.

"Her temperature is 97.2, pulse 84 and blood pressure 115/70. She is coping well with the contractions. I have been doing the breathing with her. The instruments have been boiled for five minutes and I have set up as best I can, Sister."

"Great Job Nurse Blair," said Nell. "I'll examine her now and you can do it too, if that is OK with Hazel," said Nell as she looked over towards Hazel.

Hazel was blowing out of her mouth with her lips pursed and she nodded in agreement, closing her eyes as she did so.

One thing that Hazel was good at was birthing. She was an excellent patient in labour. Nell examined Hazel and found the cervix to be four finger breadths dilated. She was in the transition phase of the second stage of labour. This baby was going to be here soon.

Nell talked the student through the vaginal exam. This was a good one for her to feel the ring of remaining cervix, the bulging bag of forewaters and, through the membranes, the sutures of the baby's head. Nell also guided Chris to assess the 'station' of the foetal head:

"This is the relationship of the level of the baby's head to the ischial spines," explained Nell.

Chris Blair was thrilled that she could feel what Nell was explaining. Chris just loved this type of work. It was so dynamic. It thrilled her and she loved the babies too.

"Would you rupture the bag of forewaters, Sister?" Chris asked.

"Good question Chris. I suppose I could do that at this stage in labour," replied Nell, "but I prefer them to rupture on their own. My personal theory is that they are a kinder dilator to the birth canal than the baby's hard head is. Only if they appear at the entroitus or if there is foetal distress will I rupture them."

Just at that moment there was a gush of fluid.

"My waters must have heard you Sister," called Hazel and they all laughed, which brought Bell running into the room to see what was happening.

"The waters have gone, Mrs. MacKinnon," informed Nell, smiling over to Bell.

"Ocht now iss that not a goo-ood sign then Sister. Is it not?" said Bell in her highland accent.

Nell noticed Chris immediately check the foetal heart and tap it out with her finger so that Nell could see the rate. Excellent Student, thought Nell, just what Miss MacGreggor said. Old MacGreggor doesn't miss a trick and sure is a great judge of character.

Hazel liked to deliver on her left side so Nell supported Hazel's leg and would conduct the delivery and talk the student through it. The second stage was longer than her last two babies were and Hazel was becoming exhausted. Nell encouraged her to relax between contractions and Bernie helped encourage her with the pushing.

Her grandma was there holding the fort. The smells of home cooking were both comforting and mouthwatering; the distinctive odour of hambone lentil soup mixed with the baker's aroma of half baked treacle scones. Nell could almost see the steam rising as the scones were buttered—day dreaming again!

Hazel's grandpa Hugh had taken the children to the adventure playground in the commodious low push chair come pram. Bessie, the one year old was sitting there bundled up like an Eskimo, and at the bottom of the pram sat wee Hugh, hugging a new red fire truck that Grandpa Brown had given him for his second birthday. Helping Great Grandpa Hugh to push the pram was Isabel who was now four years old and quite a chatterbox when her great grandpa was there. Hugh quickened their step, as it was cool in the shadow of the tenement buildings.

The MacKinnons would often take Isabel to their house for a few days to give Hazel a break, and Isobel had picked up a wee bit of the highland accent, which was lovely to hear.

She would say, "Ohh for goo-oo-dness sake," to her dolly.

They were all bonny kids when you could see their faces. Hazel's grandma had seen to that this morning. The three of them were shining and you could see to advantage their black curly hair, large brown eyes and pale skin. They were all alike, like peas in a pod. The children were warmly clad in hand knitted garments that both Bell and Hugh had knitted.

Hugh had learned to knit while he was in the merchant navy. He knitted socks, using four needles and was as fast as any knitting machine or Shetland knitter. He had once told Nell that he just kept knitting socks and each pair he made a few stitches larger to keep up with the growth of the children. Nell loved hand knitted garments.

¤

She remembered the feeling of putting on freshly knitted socks; her feet were caressed by the bounce of the stitches; the best feeling in the world!

Knitting was an integral part of Nell's family life. She and all of her sisters could knit and sew. Her father had learned to knit when he was in the Black Watch Regiment of the British Army, where they had to knit their own socks. It created good hand eye coordination and the results were useful too! She remembered her Uncle telling her that her father had run away to join the army at fifteen, saying that he was eighteen. That was in 1914, at the outbreak of the First World War.

Her father did tell them that they were sent to Russia by ship and he remembered sailing down a river in Northern Russia, which meandered through the countryside. In the distance he could see another ship that looked as if it was sailing through the fields. He said that the Russian peasants were extremely kind to them. He had talked about the peasants' homes and how they had to bring their livestock into the basement part of their homes to shelter them from the harsh conditions of the Siberian winter. That is probably why he called the coldest room in their house in Penilee Siberia, although it usually had a red adjective in front of it; "Bloody Siberia!"

Nell and her sisters learned to knit at an early age. If they needed a new jumper or cardigan they knitted it at a fraction of the cost of an inferior (or so they believed) commercially made one. They always had something on their knitting needles and used to race each other along the rows! They all sat round the fire knitting and listening to the radio.

¤

Grandpa MacKinnon arrived at the adventure playground with the children. It looked to him like a pile of junk, but was the new concept in playgrounds. He did not fancy this, so he walked on up to Eglinton Toll and along Pollokshaws Road to Queen's Park, where there was a real swing park, to his way of thinking. He had let Isobel sit on the pram, as it was a long walk for four-year-old legs, so he was pushing all three children. Hugh had been warned by Bell to stay out for the whole afternoon. She had packed him a thermos flask of hot sweet tea, and one of strained soup, a bag of buttered scones and some Farley's Rusks. He also carried the baby's bottle of milk and some orange drink. There were ample assorted cups and towels etc., and of course, they were right beside the Bluebird Café, which had the best Italian ice cream in the area. He was familiar with this spot.

The Bluebird Café held fond memories for Hugh, as he did much of his courting in this area and spent a lot of time in the Café with his various "belles", before he met the one "Bell" in his life. He took her there, too. They met in Queen's Park one Sunday afternoon when they were both listening to the band playing in the bandstand. She was there with some nurses and he was in port with the Royal Navy and was with his cousin Murdo, who lived close by in Allison Street. It is still a really nice park, thought Hugh. Well kept and well used, just as a park should be.

Hugh set up camp on a bench at the playground and let Isabel go on the merry-go-round. There was another little girl about the same age playing on it, so the speed would not be too fast. Bessie had fallen asleep, so he took wee Hugh and stood him on the merry-go- round too, tying his walking harness to the center knob that the children called 'the dumpling.'

They were grand kids, he thought. Hazel sure had her hands full though, and she did not cope very well. They probably spoiled her trying to make up for the downfalls of her mother, Lizzy. Hugh gulped hard. Better not to dwell on the subject of Lizzy. All that heartache over that would be Casanova, Donald Mac Lure. She was besought by him. She idolized him, that big idle lout. Well it's his loss. Look at the two of them there on the merry-go-round. Just looking at their happy faces did his heart good. It was really his reason for living, that, and of course Bell, who was a tower of strength. Pity she could only have the one child. If only Lizzy would come home more often and see Hazel and the children. Life has a funny old way of working itself out. I wonder what has become of Donald Mac Lure? At least Bernie Brown was a hard working lad and very fond of Hazel. Hugh continued with his thoughts.

Bernie's folk were a hard working couple. His mother Angie was a nurse at the Victoria Infirmary and his dad, Bill, was a fireman at Craigie Street Fire Station. It upset them to see the state of Hazel and Bernie's place at times. They did not visit often but instead invited Hazel and Bernie to their place in Langside, at the other side of the Park.

The Browns had two children, Bernie and Beatrice. Beatrice was married and lived in Edinburgh, so they did not see her as much as they would like. Beatrice did not have or want any children. She had three Scottie dogs, which claimed all her affection.

Hugh saw movement in the pram. Oh, wee Bessie is stirring and she will be hungry. He took wee Hugh off the merry-go-round and told Isobel to come and get something to eat in a few minutes. He was great with the children and they never gave him any hassle. They kept that for their mother. Isobel and wee Hugh sat on the park bench, beside their great grandpa, swinging their legs and tucking into a cup of warm soup in one hand and a buttered cheese scone in the other. The bench was on the road side of the swing park and they could see the pond through the trees. There were some gulps and heavy breathing coming from the pram as Jess downed her bottle. She lay back in her pram and was mesmerized by the rustling of the leaves in the tall chestnut trees above her.

Great Grandpa Hugh enjoyed his cup of tea and buttered scone too.

He said to the children, "My, that was good, was it not? A good mix… good food…fresh air and bonnie weans." He smiled at the children and they beamed back at him. The children ate everything Bell had packed. She knew them so well.

Meanwhile, back at the house, Bell had organized Hazel's kitchen and ironed everything in sight. She was there in the background, keeping the student and Nell supplied with tea and tab nabs. Hazel was having a longer time with this baby than the others. Nell checked her watch again; one-hour pushing was too long in this instance. Nell wrote down on a sheet of paper, 'delay in second stage' and Dr. Martin's phone number and the Brown's address. She gave this to Chris, the student and sent her to the Café to phone. Chris knew the Café so she hurried there—at least that phone was always working.

Nell reviewed everything in her mind; good labour, adequate pelvis as wee Hugh had been 9 pounds in weight with a good-sized head. Hazel was right on her expected date, therefore there was no post maturity factors to be concerned with, the membranes were only ruptured for a short time, therefore the risk of infection was small, the foetal heart rate good. Nell's gut feeling was that something was amiss. What was she missing? Posterior position, she thought. On the last exam she had palpated the whole anterior fontanel and there did not appear to be any moulding of the skull bones as far as she could tell. Perhaps it was just a deflexed head or a bigger baby. She had changed Hazel's position often, so once again she got Hazel on all fours.

Chris came back, followed by Dr. Martin. "Hello. Hello how are you doing Hazel?"

"Have been better Doctor," said Hazel between pushes.

Nell spoke to him and then he said, "Let's have a look at what's happening," as he prepared to examine Hazel.

"Hazel, I can see that you are getting too tired…so I will give you a hand out…OK?" Dr. Martin said quietly to Hazel, who nodded in agreement.

"I do feel a bit wabbit Doctor…it will be nice to have the baby in my arms…Oh! Ohhh…" The next contraction hit with vengeance.

"This wee one will be here soon," said Dr. Martin as he patted Hazel on the shoulder. " You are doing a good job there."

Dr. Martin took out a pair of Wrigley's birthing forceps from his bag and handed them to Nell for her to prepare them for use.

Then followed much purposeful rearranging of Hazel's position and Dr. Martin slipped the forceps' blades easily onto the baby's head and gave a steady pull, as Hazel was encouraged to push. Black hair appeared between the blades; the head was covered with a piece of the membranes.

"Oh look!" said Nell. "He has a caul." And then she was aware that a large sac was appearing behind the baby's head, an encephalocele. So that was what was causing the delay. Nell looked at Chris, the student, and saw the blood drain from the student's face.

"Nurse Blair, could you pass me that green coloured baby sheet please?" Chris looked at Nell with a glassy-eyed stare and then said, "Yes Sister, here you are," and handed the sheet to Nell. That prevented her from fainting, thought Nell.

"Well done Hazel, it is a wee boy you have." Doc Martin said, as the baby gave a shrill cry. "There is a bit of a problem with him, so he will have to go into Rotten Row's Special Care Baby Unit."

"Can we see him," Bernie said, sliding his arm round Hazel's shoulders.

"Of course you can, and you can hold him too. I will show you what we are concerned about," said Doc Martin. "I will just give him a quick exam first."

The student delivered the placenta and gave Hazel the injection of "Syntometrine" to control bleeding. She and Nell folded all the glaur away in the tarred brown paper and helped Hazel don a sanitary belt and pad.

They then placed a comfortable pad under Hazel and gave her a quick sponge down to wash off the perspiration. The warm nightie, which had been heating by the fire, warmed Hazel as Chris helped her slip it on. They worked swiftly and quietly. The baby kept letting out high pitched shrill cries that pierced the eerie silence of the room. Oh how they all longed for that lusty, gusty healthy cry of a newborn.

"What are you going to call him?" Nell asked Hazel and Bernie, trying hard to regain some normalcy to the situation.

"We thought of William, after my dad," said Bernie.

"Yes I like that," said Hazel strongly. "He is going to need all the luck of that caul to pull him through," said Hazel. "My grandpa told me that an old sailor that he knew carried a caul with him every time he went to sea."

Bell, who had been shaken by the events said, "Yes he will need that and all the love we will give him."

These mothers never failed to amaze Nell. Right after delivery they had the emotional strength of Trojans. The "caul" was supposed to be lucky and the child would never drown. Sailors, especially in the days of the sailing ships, at one time used to pay big money for cauls, which were just a primitive piece of tissue that would dry into a thin crisp. Perhaps they were not all that far off as to the usefulness of this membrane, as it has been used to help promote healing in severe burns from time to time.

They all looked at William, as Nell carefully weighed him on her spring balance scale. She lined the net with a soft baby sheet and little pillow.

"Six pounds and two ounces," Nell announced. Then she measured him. "He is nineteen and a half inches long."

The sac behind his neck was about half the size of his head. All his skull bones were present and he was moving his arms freely and sucking his right thumb. His legs lay flexed and motionless. Nell put on the cord dressing, wrapped him up in heated flannelette sheets and then a soft padded pram quilt that Bell gave her, and she handed the precious bundle to Hazel.

"Hello my wee William," she said tenderly as she placed her index finger in the clenched fingers of his left hand. "Wait till your big sisters and brother see you." She gently kissed him on the forehead and the baby's eyes looked straight up into her face.

"There you are wee man," said Bernie. "You're the greatest."

Nell signaled to Chris to come into the kitchen with her and leave them for now. Bell had tea and scones ready for them, although no one felt really ready to eat just at that moment.

"He is sucking well Sister, so is that a good sign?" Chris asked.

"Sucking is one of the five basic reflexes," answered Nell, as she sipped her tea. She wanted to say to Chris that even if there was severe brain damage, the sucking reflex would still be strong, but she could not say that with Hazel within earshot. She would have a debriefing with the student later.

"We won't know what the prognosis is till the pediatrician sees him at Rotten Row," said Nell, as she rose from the table where she had been completing the paper work and drinking a cup of tea.

"Thanks Mrs. MacKinnon, I have to make a phone call, but I will be back and we will wait with you till the ambulance comes for William. They will send out a special team for him."

On her way to the Café to phone, Nell met Hugh coming back from the park with the children. She was able to tell him about William and a wee bit of the problem.

"The children will be in time to see the baby. I know that Hazel wants that."

"Thanks Sister," Hugh said and he trudged homeward with the children all in the pram.

When Nell and Chris left the Brown's home some hours later, Bell and Hugh were in control. They had a great faith in God that would carry them through. Hazel was well cared for in bed and Hugh was reading a story from the Noddy book for Isobel and wee Hugh.

"No Gate Gampa, you've missed a bit," Isobel was heard to say.

"She knows this book inside out!" exclaimed Hugh. They all laughed. These kids will save the day for the adults in this house, thought Nell.

Bessie was in the highchair gnawing on a Farley's rusk, which was spreading over her face and bib, not to mention the tray in front of her. Bell had the place shining. Bernie had gone in the ambulance with baby William and he had phoned the fire station to pass the message on to his Dad. His parents were heading up to Rotten Row to be with him. His mother had worked with sick babies at one time, so she would ask the right kind of questions.

As Nell sat on the bus on the way home she wondered why this type of thing happened. Why three normal babies and then this? No answers came. The couple in the seat in front of Nell was having an argument about the price that the husband had paid for a bike for their son's birthday. To have an argument on a bus becomes the fellow passengers business too. There is no way that it could be done in private nor is the argument meant to be private; as if the fellow passengers were going to be judge and jury!

The wife turned to the woman across the bus from her and said, "Do you no think Ah'm right hen?"

There followed loud murmuring all over the bus about the price paid for this bike for a seven-year-old. Each passenger had a comment to make and a varying point of view.

At one time Nell heard, "Ask or Green Lady whit she thinks." Nell now belonged to this bus community.

Glasgow was wonderful for this inclusiveness. You just had to be in a bus queue and before long you knew all about the people on either side of you—where they were going and why they were going there. If there was a stranger to the city they would be given good directions and people would go out of their way to ensure that the stranger was on the correct trail.

"I'll gie yi purrich fur a month an' nae beer tae make up for it," said the would-be wounded wife.

"Gies a break hen, I thought it would be a surprise fur ye' cos ye eiy say that a never dae onythin fur him. An the wee sowel wanted a two-wheeler."

She relented, "Aw right then but in future see me first." Her position as the mainstay of the family had been momentarily threatened, but was now back on solid ground, so the rest of the bus could go home in peace, knowing that monogamous harmony ruled!

"Whit aboot the purrich an' the beer hen?"

"Acht Ah wis jist kiddin', yi big galoot!"

"Gies a wee cheeper then," and the husband kissed the wife on the cheek to a rising hum of "Aw," and "aw the nice," from the bus community.

Nell thought to herself, if they only knew about baby William Brown and the struggles that lay ahead of the wee mite, how unimportant their little episode about the bike would seem.

The three pediatricians consulted. The pediatric neurosurgeon poured over x-rays. They debated pros and cons. The baby's legs were of some concern but it was discovered that there was bilateral dislocation of both hips so that may have accounted for some of the lack of spontaneous movement. He did curl up his toes when the soles of his feet were stroked. They would require more tests to explore any other defect that baby William may have and, hopefully, they would operate in two days time. They were optimistic that the sac did not contain actual nervous tissue, but they would have to put a shunt in to drain fluid away from the brain.

The Browns stayed by William. Bernie was encouraged to go home to Hazel and let her know the score on William while his parents, Angie and Bill, would stay on for another few hours. The Nursery Sister had a great way of dealing with the families of the sick babies. She included them in all the care and dealt with the realities of each situation. That way there was no hidden agenda and the families trusted her. To understand the true situation was often a matter of coming to terms with brutal facts, and that hurt, no two ways about that.

Angie and Bill were allowed to hold William, who was laid on a pillow to support his head and the sac. They were encouraged to speak to him, sing to him, touch his hands and stroke his cheeks.

William looked up in wonderment into the eyes of the kind face of Angie Brown, who was rocking the rocking chair to and fro, singing softly.

> *"Ally bally ally bally bee*
> *Sitting on your granny's knee*
> *Looking for a wee bawbee*
> *To buy some Coulter's candy."*

She stood up and rocked him back and forth as she continued to sing.

> *"Oor wee William's*
> *Looking awfie thin*
> *A rickle o' bones covered over with skin*
> *Noo he's getting' a wee double chin*
> *Frae eatin' Coulter's candy."*

William could feel the love pouring over him and knew then he wanted to be part of this world, and his eyes, heavy with slumber, flickered, then closed. As William's eyes closed, the tears welled up in Angie's eyes. Copious tears fell. They cascaded down Angie's cheeks, almost blinding her. Bill put his arms round Angie's, supporting her and the baby, and guided her backwards towards the rocking chair. The nurse took the baby and skillfully placed him back in his incubator. Angie and Bill looked on and smiled as he pursed his lips and curled his hands under his chin. Yes the granny and grandpa were still with him; they had been there for five hours.

"And the Docs are optimistic that the operation will be successful, as far as they could tell at that stage," the night nurse said to Nell on the phone. "I think the family are just leaving now."

"Have a quiet night Nurse Porter, if that is possible with all those babies!" said Nell. "Thanks for the information. I'll call in the morning before I see Hazel, William's mother. Good night then."

Nell put the receiver back in its cradle and lay the day to rest.

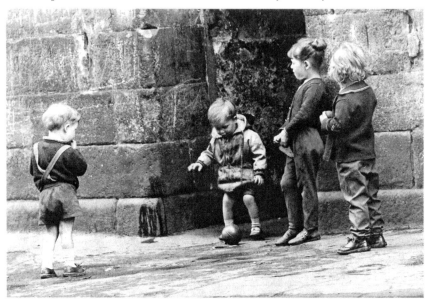

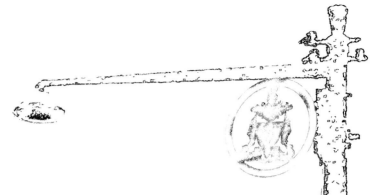

Chapter 6
Sue Taylor and Lydia Naismith

Susan Taylor was a buyer for lingerie in Watt Brothers' department store on Sauchiehall Street in Glasgow. This was a prestigious position to hold. She was thirty-five, married to George, with two teenage daughters, Christine and Fiona. They lived in Pollokshields. Lisa, George's mother, and his sister, Sammy, lived in the annex, at the side of the house, which had originally been the housekeeper's apartment.

Sammy was not the full shilling, a bit simple they say, and had never worked outside the home. She was born prematurely and had always been a bit slow. Lisa looked after Sammy well. She sheltered her and never allowed her to go to the clubs or workshops set up for the handicapped. The result of this was that Sammy was solely dependent on Lisa, who was now advancing in years. Lisa's late husband had left her with an adequate pension, but she found living beside George and Sue both comfortable and safe. She was always there to watch out for the girls if Sue was at work.

Nell called on Sue at seven in the evening to book her for a home confinement. Sue was petite, almost doll-like, with peroxide blonde hair.

"Come in Sister, it is good of you to come at this time to see me," greeted Sue and then stuck her head round a corner in the hallway towards a back living room, and called out, "Fiona tell Christine to PLEASE turn that music down for now dear."

"OK Mum," came a muffled reply through a mouth that

sounded as if it was crammed full of food.

"In here, Sister," said Sue, as she pointed to a front room just off the hallway.

Nell was aware of a figure jumping up the stairs two at a time. The sound of the Beatles'…she loves you yea yea yea…was turned up full volume, blasted for about 30 seconds and then was lowered to an almost inaudible hum. Sue had rolled her eyes upward and sucked her breath in through her clenched teeth, which were surrounded by tightened lips and her shoulders rose as if to shield her ears from the "blasted music". Her shoulders fell as the strains faded.

"Please Sister, sit down…Oh! Let me take your coat first," she added as she took Nell's coat and placed it over a beautiful Chippendale straight back dining chair which, with its twin, flanked a beautifully ornate walnut china cabinet. The cabinet almost groaned from its weighty treasures. The room was large and enhanced by the pale green and pink regency stripe wallpaper.

The ceilings were at least 14 feet high, with elaborate encrusted cornicing round the edges, echoing the feature centerpiece of a circle of roses and entwined leaves that looked down on a crystal chandelier. The ceiling was set above a deep frieze, which supported a wooden picture rail at its lowest border. There were two large pictures and one large mirror hanging from the rail. All three had deep elaborate gold coloured frames.

The modern, stark white casement sheers on the bottom half of the window sashes of the bay window, contrasted sharply with the leaded stained glass of the top sashes. The stained glass boasted the intricate Charles Rennie MacIntosh's Glasgow rose pattern in green and pink and were surrounded by dark mahogany frames that were enhanced with plush, crushed green velvet drapes, with their silken gold pull-back cords and tassels. A baby grand piano nosed its way into the bay area of the window and the gold covered dual piano stool was an elegant invitation to even the most reluctant pianist.

Nell walked towards a lounge chair to the right of the fireplace, which, surrounded by a Spanish mahogany carved mantelpiece and sides, and had become a mammoth affair. On either side of the fireplace stood matching music cabinets which were about 30 inches tall with slender Queen Anne legs, and each of the six shallow drawers could be opened by an ornate sterling silver handle that hung motionless, perfectly positioned, one above the other. The pictured tiles of the fireplace depicted a pastoral scene in light greens with pink flowers and maiden's dresses wallowing in a summer's breeze. The fireplace fender was in a highly polished brass, and at each side, incorporated a stool that had a flip lid. Atop one of these lids, propped against the downward leg of the mantelpiece, was a set of decorated bellows.

The fireplace furnishings were completed by a large bronzed companion set in the form of a knight in amour at one side and an array of hanging brass pokers and toasting forks at the other. Nell could not see the fire nest, as there was a three bar electric fire sitting rudely in front of it. The three bars were going full blast to give some instant heat. There were also hot water radiators in the room and it was a comfortable background heat. The lounge suite was a rich green floral velour with a deep cut out pattern. The carpet was a large Indian rug in light beige, pinks, greens and gold. It lay on a highly polished oak floor and feet sank noiselessly into it. This was one of the most beautiful and tastefully decorated rooms Nell had ever seen. Absolute elegant luxury! She would give her eyeteeth to be able to afford the likes of this.

Nell sat down as elegantly as she could, befitting her surroundings. She looked toward Sue, with her stark, bleached blond, brittle looking hair. She wore a black sweater that was accented at the neck with a black and tan tiger print chiffon scarf and a black, jersey wool mini skirt, which clung to whatever it touched. Black fishnet tights accented shapely legs and her worn carpet slippers seemed to shout out, "I don't belong here!"

"Sorry about that ruckus, teenagers! What more can I say?" Sue was smiling, and at the same time shrugging her shoulders and raising both palms upwards.

There was a lot that Sue could have said about her daughter, Nell sensed. Sounded like daughter Christine was proving to be a bit of a rebel at the moment. Probably had a lot to do with the pregnancy, if Nell wasn't much mistaken. Fifteen was a tricky age at the best of times, but to accept that your mother was pregnant was asking a lot! It would mean that your parents had done that ugly thing. Ugh! Perish the thought! How could they do this to Christine!

"Christine, the elder of my two daughters, is furious about this pregnancy. She told me to my face that I was disgusting and she would never speak to me again as long as she lives!" said Sue looking exasperated, shaking her head from side to side.

"Is there anything else bothering her at school?" asked Nell.

"I don't think so. She does quite well with all her subjects—about the middle of the class. She is also in one of the school hockey teams. I think that she is in the third eleven which is good for her age."

"She will come round in time. Nevertheless, it must be frustrating at the moment," said Nell empathizing with Sue. "How about your other daughter?"

"Oh Fiona, she is OK about it. She has a happy-go-lucky kind of nature. She would like a brother to boss around, she says," Sue smiled in reply.

"Fiona is the go-between at the moment, relaying messages to and fro. I really am getting tired of it and I am trying hard not to make an issue of it. I always thought that Christine was a bit more mature than this."

"She is only fifteen. This is probably the biggest adjustment that she has ever had to cope with," Nell suggested.

Nell proceeded to take Sue's maternity history. Both girls had been normal deliveries at home, in this house. In fact, Sue also had been born in this house. She told Nell that she had had a baby before she was married, a boy who had been adopted by a distant relative in England. He would be seventeen now.

"We don't talk about him. The girls know of Reginald, but don't know my connection to him. George, of course, knows the whole story," explained Sue.

"At least I know that Reginald is being well looked after and is doing well. It would have been more difficult if a stranger had adopted him and I would keep wondering how he was doing and where he was."

"I did have a miscarriage three years ago. George doesn't know about that, Sister and that confidence must be kept," Sue said in a low voice.

"Of course, Sue," reassured Nell. "Thanks for telling me as it is important, for your safety, that I know your entire obstetrical history and medical history too."

"George was having an affair with one of his fellow teachers and I found out. He finished it when I threatened to kick him out of here. You see this is my house; it was left to me by my grandmother. He was sorry for his infidelity and is still trying hard to make amends.

Things were going well again, then I went to London with some of the buyers to view a summer collection. Foolishly, I had too much to drink and a blurred one-night-stand, in revenge I suppose, and bingo, that was it. I went to see an obstetrician privately and had the operation. I was only seven weeks at the time."

"And the man, do you still see him?" asked Nell.

"No sister, he doesn't mean anything to me. I have never seen him again and I didn't even know his second name! It was an absolutely stupid, irresponsible thing to do, but it happened. It did bother me a bit to have the termination. I think that is why I wasn't too upset when I fell pregnant this time. This *is* George's baby." Sue was emphatic.

Quite the history, thought Nell, as she noted that Sue was eagerly and willingly sharing this information and, in some way, was finding it therapeutic. She was getting it out in the open for a brief moment and then could put some of it neatly back under wraps again.

Nell had just finished the full intake prenatal visit and was putting her coat on when there was a sound of car wheels crunching on the red stone chips of the driveway.

"Oh that will be George, Sister. He will drive you home."

"Hello Darling," said George, kissing Sue on the cheek.

"Good evening Sister, pleased to meet you. I'm Sue's husband, George," gushed George Taylor offering Nell an outstretched right hand.

Nell shook his hand and thought, what a limp handshake he has. So that was the high school teacher husband. He was just a bit taller than Sue, at about five feet five Nell thought. A mop of black hair sleeked back with pomade looked like an advert for Brylcream! She was not overly impressed. However, he seemed genuinely sincere when he offered to drive her home, albeit pre-planned by Sue. She did accept, as it was getting dark and the buses were few and far between at this time of night in this area.

On the car journey home George talked. He talked mostly about himself, his new car, his golf game and his admission into the tennis club.

"Are you married, Sister?" George Taylor finally asked, patting her knee and giving it a light squeeze. Nell was shocked and immediately moved her metal case to shield any further attempts of the wandering palms.

"Yes, and my husband is in the army," Nell answered. She wanted to add, "and he will have your guts for garters if you annoy me any more." She really did not like this little weasel of a man. She didn't often take a dislike to people, but there was something shifty about him. Nell was glad when she finally said, "Good night George, thanks again."

"Would you like me to see you up to your door?" George said with a nod and a wink.

"Definitely no, thanks! Your family will be waiting eagerly to see you George, I'll be fine," and with that reply, a seething Nell turned on her heels and walked briskly away. She had her door key already in her hand and was quickly inside.

What a nerve, coming on to her like that! Little sleaze ball! George Taylor was not her favourite person! Sue, on the other hand, was different to what she appeared to be.

Nell took her things off, stoked up the coal fire and made herself some Horlicks. With her hands wrapped round the generous warm steaming mug, she pondered over the evening's visit; quite the complex web we weave indeed! There must be more to the Taylor situation than meets the eye. Surely Sue must know what he is really like. What was she really like? Was she keeping a tally of tit for tat? Sue challenged Nell's value system and made her uneasy. Sue looked like a wee Glasgow hard nut, but there she was in posh surroundings with a posh accent and seemed to be genuinely nice and caring. Looks can be deceiving, never judge a book by its cover and all that jazz, but it didn't add up.

Sometimes the patients offloaded too much information onto the midwife. Nell had to do a bit of self-debriefing from some of the situations. Still she gave herself a mental reminder that she was the midwife and not some private detective. Family centered care was the buzz phrase at the moment; that's a laugh! If the furniture in that home could talk there would be some tales to tell of the last sixty years. Then again, is that not the same for any family?

It would be interesting to see how things develop. The Taylor baby was due in August so that made Sue exactly 14 weeks gestation, though Nell could not palpate the uterus above the symphysis pubis, so perhaps her dates were out. She thought too of Sue's situation, which wasn't an enviable one, even with the prestigious house full of quality furniture. It seemed to Nell that most men who have affairs can walk away from them relatively unscathed. Not so for women. Not so for Sue Taylor. She did deal with the problem as she saw it then, but it obviously still haunted her. George on the other hand, was out for all he could get. At least it certainly looked that way.

Nell's next visit to see Sue would be in four weeks. She had scheduled it for Tuesday afternoon, as that was half day closing in Glasgow. All the big stores were closed from 1 p.m. The compulsive Glasgow shoppers then streamed into Paisley, as the half-day there was a Wednesday. It was vice versa on a Wednesday for the Paisley shoppers.

With a bit of luck she wouldn't encounter the George boy. Nell rarely saw the husbands till the confinement, unless they were on shift work or unemployed or home for a specific reason. The daytime was usually the woman's domain. There were many gatherings of friends meeting or shopping that the men folk were unaware of or uninterested in. Many of the churches had Young Wives and Mothers Groups and the Catholic Church had the Union of Catholic Mothers' Group. These seemed to run in the daytime, whereas the groups for older women seemed to be held in the evening. These formal groups or informal social meetings were a Godsend to many a new mother or those who were having a difficult time in coping with varied problems. There were people to talk with who were in the same boat, coping with the same daily grind of homes and families.

There was much sharing of information and in many ways it proved to be a safety net for those feeling alienated. Sometimes Nell would be asked to be the speaker at the various meetings. She always tried to accept, with the proviso that she may be called to a confinement and they may need a plan B. It was interesting to see the natural leaders evolving in these groups.

Nell received many bookings for new patients for the summer months, especially for September. September and March were the busiest times of the year. Nine months after the Christmas and New Year festivities fell in September and March was nine months after the Glasgow Fair holiday, which was held in July. Most of the engineering works, shipbuilding, and related industries closed down for two weeks in July.

¤

The holiday dates back to 1190, by decree of William the First. The actual Fair is held on Glasgow Green, which was already a public park, then the earliest in Europe. Many of the districts in Glasgow would hold parades and fairs to mark the beginning of the holiday season. Govan always held a big fair with a Queen and four attendants picked from the local schools. People would flock to see the Govan Fair and most of the larger retail businesses would have floats. There would be daft hats and flags for sale and all the fun of the fair. Nell had a friend who stayed on Langlands Road and they had a bird's eye view of the whole parade, which would end up in Elder Park. Nine months after the Glasgow Fair was March.

¤

Nell called it the lambing season and it was about to start! This was the middle of February; Saint Valentines' day was just over. Nell had twenty bookings for March and still had six women to deliver for February. The weather was still cold, but the nights were getting a bit lighter, so that was always an indication that spring was just around the corner. Nell finished writing her notes on Sue Taylor and felt quite pleased that all her paperwork was up to date. Just then the phone rang!

"Yes? Sister Dickson here."

"Sister, it is the office here. Can you go to a confinement on London Road in Bridgeton? All the Sisters there are out. Hold on and I'll give you the information," said Miss Clarke.

"OK, Miss Clarke go ahead," said Nell grabbing a notepad and pencil.

"Mrs. Lydia Naismith, 1033 London Road, one up, middle door, she is a para three, all normal, no problems in the past. Dr. Swift is her own doctor. She is a week past her EDC. I'll send a car with one of the Student Midwives and the gas and air machine to the house, as the car can pick up Sister Syme from another confinement and take her on to another call. I will send a separate car out for you."

"Thanks Miss Clarke, it sounds as if the lambing season has started already," said Nell.

"It seems that way, Sister. Thanks, hope things go quickly for you. Cheerio for now." The phone clicked off.

Nell phoned her partner, Sister Paton.

"Hello Madge, its Nell. I have been called out to Bridgeton."

"OK, I suppose I'll be next. Is there anyone you are worried about?" asked Madge Paton, who would have to take any of Nell's patients if they went into labour.

"The only one I'm concerned about is Lillias Fleming, para two, and she is past her dates by two weeks. I saw her today and everything appeared OK, but she did have a retained placenta and a post partum hemorrhage last time. I spoke to Dr. Martin about her today and he says he will get her into Rotten Row for an induction if she does not deliver in the next 48 hours."

"Got that," said Madge. "Hope things go well tonight. Speak to you in the morning Nell."

"Fine then, I better go and not keep the car waiting. Toodlepip!" said Nell.

Nell did not mind going out to other areas of Glasgow. She worked in the South and was now going out to the East, in an old part of the city.

There was a hospital in that area called Duke Street Hospital, with an excellent midwifery department. Nell knew some of the staff there. Soon the car was speeding through Glasgow Green towards Bridgeton Cross. There were many "Crosses" in Glasgow, where two or more major roads crossed. It was usually in the centre of an area: Govan Cross, Charing Cross, Gorbals Cross, Shawlands Cross, to name but a few.

Often the Glasgow Corporation Transport System would have a time keeper's booth or "Bundy Clock" at these points. A Bundy clock was a clock into which a bus conductress would insert a time card and have the time stamped on it. There was a Bundy clock near the Southern General Hospital, where Nell did her nursing training. It was infuriating if you were short of time and the bus was ahead of time, as it would crawl along the road at a snail's pace to waste some time before stamping the card. Then the number 17 bus would speed all the way to the terminus where the driver and conductress would have their break!

The car sped on, through Glasgow Green, which was a large flat park of grass that was originally for the people of Glasgow to hang their washing up or spread the linen on it to be bleached. It was law that there could be no building on the green. At the edge of the green stands the People's Palace, a museum of every day memorabilia. The glass dome of the winter garden of the People's Palace was an inverted replica of the hull of Nelson's flagship "Victory". The people of Glasgow also honoured Lord Nelson with a monument; Nelson's column was erected on Glasgow Green long before the Nelson's column in Trafalgar Square in London was ever thought of.

¤

The word Glasgow means "dear green place", and certainly with the amount of rain and hail in the last few months, it will continue to be green, thought Nell. The river Clyde skirts the Green to the South. Nell also saw a bit of Templeton's Carpet Factory on the left with its distinctive Victorian brick façade replicating the Doges Palace in Venice. The original factory collapsed, killing 29 men, and the Glasgow City Council kept rejecting new rebuilding plans. J&J Templeton finally, in desperation, employed the services of William Leiper, an eminent architect, to find a plan that could not be rejected. Leiper's favourite building was the Doges Palace in Venice, so he replicated that to placate the Glasgow Council members. And so, the building went ahead in 1889.

Nell loved Glasgow's history, probably because she had had a Headmaster when she was in primary school, who loved to come into the classroom, much to the teacher's dismay, and tell the class stories about Glasgow and talk about the different funnels of the ships on the Clyde. The children had to "funnel spot" for him as each shipping company had different painted funnels. He was a great storyteller and Nell was a good daydreamer, so she liked when he came into the classroom.

¤

Soon Nell was passing through Bridgeton Cross, which was distinctive by the large shelter in the middle, where you could sit and wait for your tramcar to come along. The roof was shaped like an umbrella and that is what the local people called it. It was a famous meeting place. The car pulled to a halt at the close mouth at 1033 London Road. This was a very busy built-up area and the houses were of the old type of tenement with the old-fashioned coal range in the kitchen. Nell noticed that the doors on either side had bright shining brass nameplates and bell pulls. The middle door was not adorned and as the door opened, that unclean odour wafted right up Nell's nostrils.

"Ugh," she thought.

"There you are, Sister," said Willie the driver. "Here is the gas and air machine."

"Oh can you wait a wee minute Willie. I think there may be a machine here with the Student."

Nell entered the house, which was in semi darkness, lit only by the streetlights and the flicker of the fire. Being the middle flat on this level, all the windows faced the front of the building. The flat had two rooms. The toilet was on the stair landing and was shared by the families on this landing.

"Nurse did you bring a gas and air machine with you?" asked Nell peering into the kitchen.

"Yes, Sister, I'm Nurse Bette Fairly. I just arrived minutes ago," said the student midwife, moving in closer to Nell. Then in a whisper, "the electricity had been disconnected and this is my first home confinement."

"Pleased to meet you, Nurse Fairley, you will do fine," said Nell shaking Bette's hand.

"Is the electric metre just not needing some money?" suggested Nell hopefully.

"No Sister, there is no slot metre here, because I offered to put some money in," assured Bette.

"OK," said Nell, as she went to the door to speak to the driver.

"Willie can you do me a big favour?"

"Aye Sister, whit is it?" queried Willie.

"We don't have any electricity, so can you get me a dozen candles? Here is some cash and, oh, can you get me a box of matches too and if there are any fire logs—a couple of bundles? I don't know how much she has in that department but I know that your time is limited."

"Righto Sister," was the prompt reply. The drivers were not supposed to run errands, but Willie could see the bind that Nell was in.

Nell closed the door and gingerly walked back to the kitchen. She did have a small torch in her bag that would help a bit. At least there was a bit of a fire, so the place wasn't too cold.

"Hello Mrs. Naismith, I'm Sister Dickson. How are you doing?"

"Fair to middlin' I think, Sister," replied Lydia, "just caw me Lydia if you like, Sister.

"I have sent out for some candles, so we will get the place brighter soon," reassured Nell.

"Thanks Sister, we were cut aff yesterday. I sent him tae piy the bill last week and he came hame steamin' an never telt me that he hud done in aw the lolly," confessed Lydia. "Ah could o' murdered the big buggar so Ah could of."

"Well Lydia don't worry about it now, let's see how you are doing. I'll examine you and I would like Nurse Fairley to examine you too, if you don't mind?" said Nell in a calming voice.

"Aye Sister, whitever, Oh my Goad them pains ur sair," groaned Lydia.

"OK Lydia, after this pain has gone," said Nell.

"I checked the foetal heart when I got here and it was one hundred and thirty-six Sister," said Bette Fairley.

"That's good Nurse Fairley, thanks," said Nell in an encouraging manner. "We need to check it every 20 minutes or so, then after each contraction in the second stage."

"What we have to do now is assess what stage of labour Lydia in. That was a strong contraction there, Lydia, eh?" said Nell taking her hand off Lydia's abdomen where she had been assessing the strength and duration of the contraction.

Nell was aware of another few people in the house, but had not yet found out who they were. At the moment there was a woman sitting at the fire. The nurse, herself and Lydia were in the kitchen and she could hear the hum and drones of human voices from the other room. The noise did sound like someone saying, "rhubarb and ginger" over and over again. Nell had once been one of a crowd in a school play where they had to look as if they were talking to each other and had to say, "rhubarb and ginger" over and over again.

The woman at the fire answered to "Ma," when Lydia called.

"Ma will ye gie the Sister yon boax an' the ile…they're on the tap o' the wardrip in the bedroom."

"Aw right hen," said Ma, rising to go into the other room. Ma was tall and thin with black hair worn close to her head. Her overall appearance reminded Nell of Popeye's girlfriend, Olive Oyl.

Good, thought Nell, we have some supplies at least.

Nell and Bette found Lydia to be three finger-breaths dilated and a hundred percent effaced and it was definitely a head that was coming first. Nell explained to Bette what she was feeling and guided her through the internal exam.

"You are doing well. What we have been talking about means that your cervix is paper-thin and will dilate quickly, as long as you keep having strong contractions. We should have a baby here before dawn," Nell reassured Lydia.

When the driver brought Nell the candles and logs, it was ten thirty and all was well.

"Put a couple of candles in front of that mirror," said Nell to Bette, "a couple over there and again about here."

There was now a circle of light round the side of the bed in the bed recess and from the fire too. The fire was burning fiercely now, with a couple of logs, and Danny Naismith made a brief appearance with a shovelful of coal dross from the inside bunker, to augment the fuel. He muttered something about there was too much coal dross in a bag of coal. Nell felt that too when she got her coal delivered. She always had to clear the dross out the coal bunker.

¤

She recalled the time that she was doing that job and was covered in coal dust from head to toe when she was called out to a confinement. She had a quick bath and mistakenly put "pretty feet" under her arms instead of deodorant. She had to start again and get it all washed off. She had visions of her arms falling off as the "pretty feet" was to get rid of hard skin! The car was at the door waiting on her! Her oxters burned for days!

¤

In the candlelight Nell, could now see more of Lydia. She was of the same mould as her mother; a sort of Olive Oil mould, but Danny was no Popeye. He was tall and lean. Lydia's face was weary looking and she had dark circles under her eyes and a front tooth missing.

"Olive, sorry,…I mean Lydia, you might be better to walk around for a bit," said Nell blushing at her mistake. In the not too bright room no one noticed.

Nell set Bette to walk with Lydia and time her contractions and take the foetal heart rate every fifteen to twenty minutes.

"I'll go aroond the hoose," said Lydia.

"Here take a couple of candles with you," said Nell, handing the candles and the box of matches to Bette.

"Ta," said Lydia spontaneously. "The wee yins don't know whit's goan own, an he's no much help either, but ma Da's wi them an he likes to tell the weans stories."

That accounted for the rhubarb and ginger tones. Nell went down to the phone box to let Dr. Swift know that Lydia was in labour.

"Thanks Sister. Do let me know if you need me, otherwise, I will call in and see her in the morning. She looked a bit pale when I saw her a couple of days ago, but her hemoglobin is 11.2, so don't worry on that score," reassured Dr. Swift.

"Thanks doctor, I'll tell her that you will be in to see her in the morning. Good night."

When Nell got back, she checked with Bette and then set out to get things ready for the baby. The maternity box consisted of the oil Ma had produced and a tatty leather case. Inside was the sum total of Lydia's nest making preparations: a pair of flannelette sheets in a brilliant pink, a hot water bottle, an array of new and old baby clothes, a well washed knitted shawl, some baby blankets, flannelette baby wraps, baby soap and baby powder. She also had a little bottle of surgical spirit for the cord. She probably had to hide the stuff from Danny or it would end up in the pawnshop.

Nell looked about in vain for a cot or pram to put the baby in then said, "Lydia do you have a cot or a pram for the baby?"

"Aye Ah hud a nice wee carry-cot wi'wheels, that a wummin frae the church gied me, bit he took it awe tae the pawn shoap fur lolly fur fags. I'll get it back oot oan Tuesday, when ah get ma family allowance."

"We can use one of these drawers till then," said Nell in a matter of fact way, not to make a great deal out of the pawnshop visit. The drawer was just perfect. It was a half drawer of about thirty inches long and was deep so it made a snug bed.

"I'll pit it at the back o' the bed," said Lydia smiling. She was relieved that Nell understood the way things were, as she once had a Sister who would "tut tut" about everything that did not please her. Round the fire stood a big fireguard on which Nell hung the baby clothes to air and heat.

The hours passed. The candles flickered. The fire crackled. The labour progressed. The women blethered. The foetal heart rate was recorded. The gas and air machine valve flapped.

Finally at 3:33 a.m., with a wail from Lydia, a tear from Bette, a sigh of relief from Nell and an "Oh my Goad" from Ma, wee Lydia the second gave a gasp and a cry as she was born onto her mother's abdomen by candlelight.

"Good job, Nurse Fairley," Nell said, still with the Dee Lee suction apparatus in her mouth, after aspirating the baby's nose and mouth. "Use the cotton wool to dry the baby's eyes. Take your time, there is no rush now and clamp the cord in two places and cut the cord between the clamps. That's the way, good! Now dry the baby with the terry nappy—here is the warm wrap for the wee cherub. Now give her to her mum, she will keep her warm while we do the rest."

Nell liked to talk the students through the first couple of home deliveries, as it was different from the hospital. She wanted them to feel confident in what they were doing so that the experience would be positive. Nell never relaxed till the placenta was delivered and the mother was in a stable and safe state with minimal bleeding. Everything went well here and Danny came in to say hello to his first daughter, wee Lydia. He seemed quite concerned for both mother and daughter; but the two boys were still fast asleep. They would see their new sister in the morning. Danny took the baby in his arms and swayed her to and fro and said, "Am yir daddy hen, yir stuck wi' me, an' jist wait till yir big brothers see you!"

There was nothing like a home confinement to bring out the best in everyone. It was certainly a perpetual miracle and Nell always thanked God each and every time, without fail. She was always awed and humbled by the experience.

Just as the baby was being dressed, after her bath, Ma produced a pink knitted matinee jacket with hat, bootees and mitts to match.

"I was hoping it wid be a wee lassie this time sister," Ma said with a grin like a Cheshire cat on her face. "Ma auld neighbour knitted these, so she did, for Ah canny knit."

And so the pink bundle, in her special knitted layette, was placed in the heated pink flannelette sheet and then into the drawer at the back of the bed in the bed recess. Wee Lydia Naismith set out on life's journey, like another 90 babies that night in the City of Glasgow with a warm welcome to the "Dear Green Place."

"The cor's here sister," informed Danny.

Nell buttoned up her double breasted coat, slipped the green belt through the green bakelite buckle and tugged to tighten it, lifted her case and with the student in tow bid farewell to the Naismiths.

As they climbed into the corporation car at 4:15 a.m. Nell and Bette were tired, but relieved that all had gone well. The streetlights seemed so bright compared to the candlelight of the night.

"Well that is a good one for your blue book," said Nell to Bette.

The blue book was a journal that the student midwives had to keep of ten home confinements that they attended.

"Yes Sister, that will be the first and have pride of place," agreed Bette.

"Sister, why do these women stay with these men in these conditions?" asked Bette.

"That's a loaded question," answered Nell and went on. "The women are very loyal to their men. I once tried to suggest to one woman that she should report her husband for cruelty, but she turned on me and defended him. She said that she had provoked him into a temper. Often they are trapped, though, or just going through a rough patch. We have got to remember that we are only getting a snapshot of their life. We really never know the whole story. Many of them, given half a chance, could become independent in their own right."

"I am definitely going to be independent," said Bette Fairley firmly.

"I think every woman should have the capability to be independent if she needs to be," said Nell, as the car sped through the sleeping Glasgow streets.

"Well you sure can travel all over the world with Scottish nursing qualifications and midwifery," added Bette as she looked intently out of the window.

Nell loved going through Glasgow at this hour of the morning. The streets were almost deserted except for the bakers and newspaper workers going to and coming from work.

"Drop the student off first at Ingram Street please Dave, before you take me home, and she can take in the gas and air machine and the notification of birth form for me," requested Nell.

"Right you are, Sister," said Dave the driver.

"Thanks Nurse Fairley, you did well," said Nell as Bette got out of the car. "Hope to see you again."

"Thanks Sister for everything," said Bette.

The student midwives had a tough time, thought Nell. She remembered it well; they had to attend lectures whether they were out all night or not. Still, she mused, she, herself, would have to do her mornings work before she could get a decent rest. So it is good training for them!

Back home, Nell set her alarm clock for eight o'clock. That would give her an hour or so. It was just as if she had blinked when the "Bell from Hell" sounded in her ears. She shot off the bed stunned…and wondered where she was. Slowly she focused back to the present and phoned Madge.

"Just got back before six, did any of my patients phone?"

"Just one false labour—Mrs. Jones. Give me a few of your visits so that you can get home early for a sleep," Madge offered.

"I'll give you two that are close together and that would help a great deal. Thanks a million," Nell said gratefully.

It was good the way that they were able to help each other. Nell was tired and would welcome her bed at the end of the morning visits. She repacked her confinement case, ready for the next miracle.

Nell enjoyed a cup of tea and a slice of toast with marmalade to ease her back into the regular morning mode. Then she buttoned up her green double breasted coat and slid the green belt through the green bakelite buckle and tugged to tighten it and with case in hand, left for her morning visits.

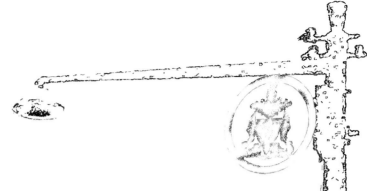

Chapter 7
Lillias Fleming

"Big breath in—good—hold it—pushdown, long and hard—great work Lillias. Let it out, that's the way, and again big breath in—hold it and push down, great pushing."

"Sister can you see any ting yet?" Lillias uttered in her soft Dublin accent as she recovered between contractions.

"Yes," said Nell, "in the distance there is a wee bit of head. I see more when you push, you are doing well!"

Nell used a cool damp cloth to mop the perspiration from Lillias' brow and swept her blonde hair away from her temples and the back of her neck, as she was feeling the heat of the labour. It was hard work, this labour, and well named!

"Why does the baby keep going back?" asked Lillias.

"Well, the contraction pushes the baby down and when it wears off the pelvic floor muscles recoil and the baby's head slips back, but it rotates into a better position as it does so. Each time it makes a wee bit of progress. That way, the birth canal opens gradually," said Nell, slowly giving Lillias a bit of shoulder massage in an effort to relax her tense muscles.

"Just try and sink through the bed Lillias, that's the way, be a rag doll—great stuff."

"Oh! Oh! Here it comes again!" said Lillias quickly.

"Deep breath in through your nose, hold it and push 2–3–4–5–6–7–8—let it out. Big breath in again, hold it push 2–3–4–5–6–7–8—let it out. And big breath in again push 2–3–4–5–6–7–8—let it go and relax. Jimmy a sip of water for her," and Nell nodded to Jimmy as she wrung out a cool wet face cloth to sooth Lillias' brow, temple and neck once more.

"That's the way—you are relaxing better now." Nell checked the foetal heart rate. "Everything is tickity-boo in there, and in fact it sounds like galloping horses!" Nell smiled at Lillias and Jimmy and they returned relieved grins.

An hour earlier, when Nell arrived at the Fleming's apartment, Lillias was literally climbing the walls. Nell heard the screams as she entered the close mouth.

Sounds like she is in transition, thought Nell. This should not take long. The neighbours were out on the stair head landings, alarmed and discussing the noise. One older woman, standing in her doorway, said to Nell as she past, "Sister, I have a phone if you need it hen."

"Thanks, Mrs. Dick?" said Nell, looking at the gleaming nameplate at the side of the door.

She nodded in recognition of her name and smiled.

"These lassies have their work cut out for them," said Mrs. Dick with her arms folded, moving her elbows from side to side till her crossed forearms came to rest under her bulging floral apron with the frilled shoulder straps.

As Nell made her way up the stairs, she heard a few horrifying birthing stories being graphically told. Words such as "double breech", "double pneumonia", "rupture", "twilight sleep", "big heed" and "touch and go", told her that the "stair heed gossip" had a full head of steam and probably would keep going till the Fleming baby was delivered. The Flemings lived on the top floor. Nell kept climbing.

Two of the neighbours had gone to Lillias' aid and were trying their best to help calm her down. Jimmy was as frantic as she was. He had never seen her in such pain and felt utterly helpless and believed without a doubt that there was something drastically wrong.

Nell soon gave them all jobs to do while she spent time alone with Lillias. Within ten minutes, things were under control. She always believed that pain is what the patient says it is. Lillias was too far on in labour to get any injectable pain medication, as it would affect the baby's breathing. She could have the gas and air if she wanted it and Nell had it ready for use, but Lillias did not fancy putting the black mask over her face, as it reminded her of an ordeal at the dentist's. However, she was doing fine now that she had gotten a handle on the contractions.

Nell reinforced with her that it was mind over matter. She was in second stage of labour and did not have to bear the pain any more, as she could push with it. She was in control as she said, "Here we go again," and took a big breath in and held it. This time Jimmy Fleming did the counting, as Nell had encouraged him to do.

The doorbell rang and the student midwife arrived. It was Nurse Fairley again and she was pleased to see Nell.

"Good timing Nurse, this is Lillias and Jimmy Fleming, having their second baby. They have a little boy of two so this is to be the pink bundle. Dad wants a daughter this time." Nell had got Jimmy involved. Lillias had told her that last time he sat through in the kitchen as the midwife said he would just get in the way, so she did not want him in the room. Nell liked to get the dads involved and it was good to have another pair of hands too.

"Hello Mr. and Mrs. Fleming, I'm Bette Fairley, the student midwife and I'm so pleased to be sharing this with you. Thank you."

Nell thought, that was a nice way of putting it Bette. She will do well with her friendly approach.

"Jimmy is doing well with the coaching, nurse and Lillias is pushing like a Trojan so, check the foetal heart rate after each contraction and you can use this basin here for the face cloth." Nell liked to get everyone knowing what they were doing.

The Flemings were an interesting couple. Lillias was from Dublin and had come over to Glasgow to study art at Glasgow School of Art, where she met Jimmy. He also was studying there, specializing in photography. Together they opened a Photographer's Studio in Victoria Road. To augment the business they sold artwork and framed pictures. Their business was just beginning to pay for itself. Jimmy was from Glasgow and his parents gave them a hand with baby sitting wee Sean. They had come early this morning and took Sean "out of the way", as they put it.

"Do you have names picked out?" asked Bette.

"Only girl's names: Yvonne or Bridget. Jimmy is determined that this baby is a girl. He wants to dress her up like a doll in pink frills. In fact, he has even bought a little dress and frilly pants," Lillias said, smiling.

Bette was a bit troubled about this declaration and thought that she better not pursue it further. There was an awkward silence, which was broken by Lillias saying, "Here we go again."

They all took up their positions for pushing: Nell and the nurse at each side and Jimmy beside Lillias counting for her, as she pushed three times.

"Great Lillias, the head is staying there this time and you may feel a sort of burning. Just breathe easily now. During the next contraction we may ask you to stop pushing and pant instead as the baby's head is born," said Nell in a calm reassuring voice, looking right into Lillias' eyes.

"OK Sister, it is stinging a bit," said Lillias, as she looked up into Jimmy's eyes. Jimmy had his right arm round her shoulders and was holding her left hand in his.

"Now Nurse, let the baby's head push against the fingers of your left hand. That way you will help increase flexion so that the vertex will emerge. When you feel that your fingers cannot stretch over the head any further, that is crowning, the biparietal eminences will stretch your hand to the full. At that time, tell Lillias to pant. The force of the contraction will deliver the baby's head probably with this contraction or the next. Continue to guard the perineum with your right hand and the pad." Nell spoke clearly and calmly to Bette who was nodding in reply to the various instructions.

There was hardly a sound during the next contraction save for Bette saying, "pant Lillias," and Lillias' expiring through her mouth, "Haa!—haa!—haa!—haa!—haa!—oooooh!" The latter changed into a low guttural moan as the head was born. It was a big head.

"Well done Lillias, and beautifully controlled, Nurse," said Nell as she watched Bette clean the baby's eyes while she did a little aspiration of secretions from the baby's mouth and nose with the Dee Lee suction catheter. The bluish coloured head sat there facing the inside of Lillias' right thigh.

It was always a surreal moment with the head born before the birth of the baby's body, Nell thought, suspended animation of sorts.

Nell suddenly noticed Jimmy's face staring at the baby's head and his face becoming ashen.

"Jimmy!" called Nell in a demanding way, and he looked directly at her, "The heart rate is good and the baby is good. You are doing a great coaching job. Lillias you can give a push with the next pain if you feel you must." The colour flushed back into Jimmy's face and he was back on track.

"The baby will be born with the next contraction. Chin and occiput grip Nurse, good—Nurse, down to the bed—anterior shoulder. Now watch the perineum as the other shoulder is born, complete the curve on to Mum's abdomen—that's the way great!"

An almighty wail was uttered by Lillias' second son.

"It's a big boy," said Nell and in the same breath through the baby's lusty cry she asked, "Jimmy will you cut the cord for us?"

"Sure Sister, what do I do?"

"Here you are—take these—cut hard just here—that's the way—great—thanks Jimmy."

"Congratulations to you both—he doesn't look like a Bridget or an Yvonne, but he is a beautiful big baby boy," said Nell, smiling.

No one could deny that. He had pinked up as he immediately as he started crying and he had shoulders on him like a wrestler.

"Look at those legs," said Nell. "He has good knees for a kilt!" They all laughed!

"He could wear a few different tartans," said Jimmy "even the Irish kilt." "He is much bigger than Sean was and has a good pair of lungs!" Jimmy continued, smiling down at him. "You're a wee smasher! Thanks Darlin', that was quite an ordeal for you", and he bent down and kissed both Lillias and the baby.

"He looks like Jimmy—I think we will call him James!" said Lillias, "Yes, how about James Kelly Fleming? Kelly is my maiden name you know. What do you think Jimmy?"

"I think it suits him right down to the ground. JK it is," said Jimmy grinning. "We're about to rename the business. I think it will be "J and L Fleming and Sons". That has a great ring to it.

Nell was pleased to hear this, as Jimmy had his heart set on a girl. She heard him on the phone later saying, "No I'm not disappointed in the least, and I cut the cord! No bother, you just cut between the clamps…" at this comment Nell winked at Bette who smiled knowingly back at her.

Everything Nell and Bette had to do was done and James was busy breastfeeding, when Dr. Cairns called into see how things were going.

"You ladies can certainly get things going," he addressed Lillias.

"Oh Doctor, it was really fast and furious this time, so unlike the first," Lillias replied.

"Second babies are often like that m'dear. Now keep on with the pregnancy vitamins and iron supplement for now and I'll be in to see you tomorrow. Sister will tell you about the after pains and what to do about them, as you don't have them with a first baby either," Doc Cairns said before he left the room. He congratulated Jimmy in the hallway on his way out.

"A corporation car will pick up the gas and air machine sometime in the afternoon and we will be back in to see you before 5 p.m.," said Nell before she and Bette left to catch up on the morning's work.

"That was a good idea to get the father involved, Sister. Did you know that it was going to be a boy?" asked Bette as they headed down the stairs.

"I knew there was a 50/50 chance," said Nell. "I always try to encourage the dads to be part of the delivery, but some of them are terrified. That's why I give them a specific task to do. If they are busy doing something then they don't dwell on the actual pain that their wife is experiencing. Seeing someone you love in pain and not being able to alleviate it is frightening."

Nell smiled at the neighbours on the way down the stairs. They had already heard the news and Nell knew that there would be pots of soup and home baked scones making tracks up those stairs before very long.

Out on Pollokshaws Road the wind was picking up, but it was dry. The visits Nell had to do were in clusters, so that was good, and with Bette to help her, they could soon whip round them in no time at all. She did want to do a prenatal visit on Sue Taylor prior to going back to check on Lillias on her homeward journey. Nell kept looking for a bus, but they kept walking. Sometimes the buses were few and far between. It was warmer to walk. She knew that the bus would stop for her between stops anyway, so on they walked.

Sue Taylor was really pleased to see her and greeted her with, "Sister you are a sight for sore eyes, I was just thinking of you this very moment."

"I know that I am a week ahead for our arranged visit, but I was passing your door and it is Tuesday, your half-day off, so I thought I would try and see if you were in," explained Nell.

"Sister I desperately need to talk to you. I was going to phone you," Sue said with urgency in her voice.

"What is the matter Sue?" asked Nell, as she and the nurse followed Sue into her back room, which was a large living room with a kitchenette off it leading to the back door and porch. Everything shuddered suddenly as a heavy goods train trundled by on the railway at the bottom of the sloping garden.

When the three women sat down, Sue began. "I really don't know where to start Sister," Sue said as she squeezed the fingers of one hand through the fingers of the other hand.

"Sue, just start at the beginning. I will help if I can," said Nell in a reassuring manner, laying her hand on Sue's arm as she spoke.

"Well Sister, it's about my daughter Christine's friend, Jenny. I think she is being sexually abused by her father and elder brother. I may be wrong, but I am 99% sure. She comes here a lot with Christine, especially on her way home from hockey practice at Norwood on Dumbreck Rd. She is a nice girl and her mother died when she was twelve, just over three years ago. She does the cooking and they have a housekeeper and a few days a week her father has to travel with his job."

"Does she have any siblings?" asked Nell softly.

"She has three older brothers; the eldest is in the Royal Navy, one is at College and the other one is still at school," answered Sue.

"What did she tell you, Sue?" speared Nell.

"That's it Sister, she really didn't directly tell me anything. That's what's been troubling me. I keep saying to myself that I just imagined it," hesitated Sue.

"Sue, you wouldn't be so upset if there wasn't cause for concern. Tell me what made you suspect that Jenny is being abused," Nell said, leaning forward towards Sue.

"When I got back from doing some shopping I had bought four packets of sanitary napkins, as they were on sale at Boots. When I was taking them out of my shopping bag Jenny said, "Oh I need to buy more of them as I have to wear them all the time, especially with my brother and Dad home together."

You could have knocked me down with a feather! So I asked her if she had a discharge, and she said yes and that she was all sore down there." Sue heaved a sigh of relief.

"Well you are not imagining anything Sue. At least Jenny needs some treatment, as it sounds like this lassie has a venereal disease," affirmed Nell.

"I told her to go to her doctor and tell him," said Sue, "but she said that she was too embarrassed to do that. So then I thought that you may know a lady doctor for her."

"Sue, this is serious, you know. We have to get this girl into a safe place. If her father and brother are abusing her, they will end up in jail." Then Nell went on. "We have to deal with this very sensitively. I will get an appointment for her to see Dr. Jane Sear, who is a public health doctor, and she is a wonderful woman. She will also be the best one to deal with the legalities."

"Jenny will be here soon with Christine, as they have hockey practice today," said Sue.

"Good. Lets strike while the iron is hot," said Nell decisively. "Can I make a few phone calls, Sue?" asked Nell.

"Please do Sister; I'm relieved that something is going to be done about this. I wouldn't let Christine go to Jenny's place and I tried to speak to Christine about it, but of course I am not in her good books at present, so it has been difficult. I tried to speak to my husband, George, about it and he said it was none of my business and I was probably jumping to the wrong conclusions." Sue heaved a sigh of relief and said to Bette, "How about a wee cup of tea?"

¤

Christine Taylor was furious with her mother. It was three days since her mother behaved so secretively and got Jenny to see the Green Lady and then the car came and took Jenny away to see a doctor. What was all the fuss about anyway? Since her mother had become pregnant she was really weird. Pregnant at her age…it was really disgusting! Christine had not seen Jenny since. Her brother wasn't at school either. What was happening? She was determined to have it out with her mother when she came home from work today. She was lost without Jenny. One of the teachers said that Jenny might not be back to school ever. Her mother really was a piece of work.

Sue came home from work. She looked tired. She had had some abdominal pain all afternoon. Must have been that chicken curry she ate last night. She should leave off the spicy things till after the baby, but she did enjoy it—and the evening out with George. She was relieved too, that Jenny had been taken into care while an investigation was underway. If only she could speak to Christine. She should try tonight. After all she is her mother.

Sue flopped into a chair in the back room and kicked off her shoes. That pain was piercing. It was definitely getting worse.

"Go and get your gran, Christine. I don't feel good," Sue tried to shout breathing in deeply after each word. Christine was about to give her a snide comment about not speaking to her, when she looked over at Sue and saw that her mother was far from well. She saw dark circles round her eyes and a bluish ring round her mouth.

"OK Mum!" and she disappeared out the door to return moments later with her gran in tow.

"I think that you better call an ambulance, I think I have appendicitis.

Oh God! Oh God! The pain is awful!" moaned Sue as she rolled over on the couch crumpling into the foetal position.

Christine got the phone number for her gran and ran and got the tartan travel rug to put over her Mum. She propped a cushion under her mum's head and stroked her forehead with her hand as she said, "You will be OK Mum. The ambulance will be here soon. I'll come with you to the hospital as gran better stay here and try to get a hold of Dad."

Sue looked up at Christine and thought, well, she is in control of the situation, good for her taking charge. Then another wave of pain gripped her tight and she swooned under it.

It had only been an hour. It felt like days. Christine was still in the waiting room of the Samaritan Hospital for Women. She had phoned her gran to say that they were taking her mother to the operating theatre, but where was her Dad? She had read all the posters on the wall about vaccination, home safety, hand washing and head lice, but still the image of her mother's ashen face as they wheeled her away was vividly imprinted in her mind's eye. Was her Mum going to die? Her eyes welled up with tears as she hugged herself and rocked to and fro on the chair with her head bowed into her crossed arms. Suddenly she felt someone touch on her shoulder.

"Dad!" she cried, but when she looked up, it was her friend Jenny leaning over her. "Jenny what are you doing here?" asked Christine, surprised.

"I'm in here as a patient Christine," said Jenny quietly. "It's a long story and I want to tell you one day. You are my best friend."

"Was it my Mum that caused you to be in here Jenny?" asked Christine with tears running over her cheeks.

"Well yes, in a way, she did," admitted Jenny, "but she was only thinking about me and what was best for me, do believe that please?"

Christine pleaded, "Why are you here Jenny?"

"No one was supposed to know where I am."

"My Mum collapsed with terrible pain and she thought it was her appendix. She looked like death and they have taken her to the operating theatre just now. They said something about an ectopic pregnancy, what ever that may be. I thought that you were my Dad, I am waiting on him. My gran was trying to locate him."

"I better get back to my ward, the Sister let me go to the shop for these magazines. I'll try and see your mum later. The night nurse is nice and she may let me visit her."

The two girls hugged each other and Jenny left. Christine watched her as she walked back along the corridor in her pale pink fur trimmed slippers and dusty pink candlewick dressing gown. She had the magazines under her left arm. She wondered what the whole story was; she knew that it was serious whatever it was. The corridor was long and Jenny looked like a six-inch doll before she made a right turn and disappeared.

Where is Dad? thought Christine. I hope he isn't messing about with that floozy Patsy Orr, the arty-farty teacher, again.

She had once overheard her mother calling Patsy a "nympho" and not knowing what it meant she looked it up in the Oxford dictionary. It read, "nymphomania; *morbid and uncontrollable sexual desire in women*." She did not like Patsy. Liberal art she taught indeed! She was too liberal with Dad. I'm glad she moved away to Hyndland School; a good place for her; as far away from her weak Dad as possible!

At that very moment, her Dad and Patsy sat across the table from one another at the meeting, their eyes meeting too often. He could not take his eyes off of her and she knew it too and gave him sensual glances from time to time. She left as soon as the meeting was over, slipping a piece of paper into his pocket as she brushed passed him. He had to stay to discuss an item with the chairperson.

He finally got into his car and was homeward bound when he took the note from his pocket.

It read, "Coffee will be ready, please come."

His heart raced a bit and he was annoyed that it did. He had had a good night with Sue last night; they discussed Christine's future. She wanted to be a nurse and go into Logan and Johnston pre-nursing college. She could go there when she was seventeen and that was only fourteen months away. He was a father and had responsibilities, even a new baby on the way, so why did a few words on a scrap of paper fill him with excitement? His "Ego and Id" were warring, as Sigmund Freud would say. He had finished the affair with Patsy seven months ago. He really had nothing to say to her; he didn't even like coffee! He knew only too well that there would be more than coffee on the menu.

He swithered momentarily, but somehow his car headed away from home and towards the offered coffee. Havelock Street, the road sign said, and in his subconscious he heard Sue saying, "That one needs to HAVE LOCKS on her knickers".

Still, visions of Patsy outdid Sue's warnings and filled his senses. He pulled his car to a halt as his heart began to race and his mouth became a little dry. Up the stairs he went like a teenager, two at a time with a spring in his step and as he put his hand up to knock the door, he almost fell in because she opened it at that precise moment.

Patsy caught hold of his Glasgow Boys High School tie and as she pulled it off, she pulled him to her. His jacket fell to the floor, on top of his tie, followed by his shirt. She was kissing him with urgency and he responded with an awakened pent up passion of the last months. She was red hot; dressed in a silky red negligee with matching high heeled mules which were adorned with cluster of feathers that fondled her toes as she walked backwards to the bedroom. Soon they were wrapped in each other's arms, their naked bodies heaving in love making rhythm.

"You have to leave Sue. She can't give you what I am giving you, Georgie Porgie."

Patsy was whispering in George's ear as she clung to him like a limpet. A few moments of climax and George lay back on the bed. She was immediately on him again. She has such a sexual appetite, thought George. It was wonderful!

"I have to make the most of you when I see you," she smiled, as she poured massage oil all over him.

"Hey! You might have heated that a bit Patsy my girl, you don't want to give your lover a shock now do you?" George pouted as he wallowed in oil and attention.

Patsy was twenty-eight, seven years younger that George, and had been divorced from her abusive husband for two years. During the separation, she had confided in George that she was having a hard time adjusting, and George helped her move into her apartment. They had had a brief affair that Sue found out about and he had broken it off. Patsy then moved schools and for a while they did not see each other. Lately they had both been on a committee for an upcoming exhibition and he had resisted the old embers trying to ignite again, until today.

Today it had been unbelievable, better than ever. He must be one of the best lovers in Glasgow, thought George, as the little man syndrome boosted his already inflated ego. He should really divorce Sue and come home to red-hot Patsy every day. Better wait till after the baby though. If only the house was in joint names. That would give him a bit of collateral. He must have another try to put the house in joint names. It would take a lot of sweet-talking but he would get round Sue in the end.

¤

"Where the Hell have you been, George Taylor?" screamed his mother as he came whistling through the front door of his home.

"Hold on now," replied George with both hands up on either side of his face. "I have been to a meeting at the University Library, and the traffic was murder."

"That meeting was over three hours ago. We have been trying to get a hold of you! Sue has a ruptured ectopic pregnancy and is at death's door and Christine, the wee soul, is waiting for you at the Samaritan Hospital."

Lisa was looking at him with an all knowing eye and sniffing him out.

She said, "You can't fool me George. Remember that I had a life of the same with your father. I know that you have been with a woman this afternoon; I can read you like a book. No matter who she is, she will never be half the woman that Sue is. Now get to that hospital before I take my hand across your face and don't think that I couldn't do it. I'm still your mother!"

George ducked as if to avoid his mother's hand and scurried out of the house into the car and zoomed away at top speed. His heart was racing for the second time today, but for a very different reason.

He saw Christine in the waiting room. "Christine! Christine! It's me," he called to her.

Her tear stained face turned towards him and through glassy reddened eyes she saw him and nodded in recognition, but she had no energy to elicit a welcome. She sat there slumped in a chair.

"What is happening, Christine dear?" he asked tentatively.

"The doctors have been asking for you for ages. Mum is very ill and they may try to move her to the Victoria or the Royal for intensive care. She might die," said Christine in a strange monotone voice that lacked her usual luster and vitality.

George looked at his daughter and a lump came to his throat. He gulped and asked quietly, "Where do I go to see the doctors?"

"Just there," said Christine pointing to a door that had a "PRIVATE" sign on it and George immediately walked towards it.

¤

"Hello Mum, how are you doing?" said Fiona Taylor and she walked into her Mum's hospital room, "Christine will be here shortly, she is just speaking to Jenny."

"Hello darlin' it is good to see you. I have missed you. How's gran holding out?" asked Sue.

"She is fine. Christine and I are doing most of the cooking. We let her tell us what to do. She will be in to see you tonight," said Fiona breezily.

Sue thought, what great girls I have. They are so sensitive and kind.

"It is good of the sister to allow you in to see me. She said, as it is a single room no one would make a fuss. Under the age of sixteen you can't visit during the week," said Sue.

"Do you not think that I look sixteen?" asked Fiona, sticking her chest out, then she looked at her mother and they both burst out laughing!

It was good for Sue to laugh. She had come very near to death, they told her, but she had responded well to the blood transfusions and they did not need to move her from the Samaritan Hospital for women. Sue was pleased about this as it made it easier for people to visit.

George would be coming tonight. She was really disappointed with him, as she noticed he had some tell tale scratches on the side of his neck. She had noticed them and the distinctive perfume of "Chanel No 5" when he had bent down to kiss her that first day after the operation. She had seen and smelled the like before, when he was having the affair with Patsy. The scratches were from her long witch-like nails.

So it's on again with Patsy, Sue thought to herself. Oh well! She would deal with him once and for all when she got stronger. Her daughters were just wonderful and at least he had left them alone, not like Jenny's father.

She smiled at Fiona and wondered how Jenny was doing. Poor wee thing she was, having her childhood torn from her. The bastards! Just then, Christine came in with flowers and broke her mother's train of thought.

"I have fresh cream meringues from the City Bakery for you, Mum. How's it going? You look much better now. More like your old self." said Christine.

"I'm feeling a wee bit stronger every day," reassured Sue. "I hope to be home to recuperate in a few days. Tell me now, what has been happening at school?"

The two Taylor girls chatted non-stop for the entire visiting hour. Even after the bell rang to announce the close of visiting, Fiona came running back because she had forgotten to tell her mother something! Sue was pleasantly tired after the visit, and she nestled into her pillows and fell soundly asleep. Life would be intolerable without her girls. She loved them very much.

At the evening visiting, George and his mother arrived. Sue chatted with Lisa but had no conversation for George. The very sight of him offended her, like a knife twisting in her gut.

A week later, Sue was home. It felt wonderful to walk through the house again. She could feel her mother's and her grandmother's presence in the front room, where she had requested the coal fire to be lit. She rested there, with lots of pleasant memories to keep her company. George came home from work and came in to see her.

"Oh! You are in here darling," said George surprised to see the fire lit and Sue lying on the couch beneath an eiderdown quilt.

"Yes," said Sue with an edge to her voice, "and why shouldn't I be?"

"You don't normally sit through here on your own," George was forced to reply.

"Well these are not normal circumstances, are they George?" queried Sue.

George looked at her and strangely, he felt his stomach churn.

Sue looked George straight in the eye and said, "I will give you two hours to get you and your miserable belongings out of my house. Your mother and sister can stay on as long as they want to. My lawyer will be serving you separation papers next week and I gave him the Havelock Street address. The girls are fully aware of the situation."

"You can't be serious Sue. You need me here to help you recover; you are not in a fit state to make this kind of decision. You have been through a rough time; you are not in your right mind," stumbled George as he strutted about the room.

"How dare you accuse me of not being in my right mind! I am not the unfaithful partner here. While I was fighting for my life, you were with her. I could smell her fancy perfume off you as you bent over me. You disgust me. Now go and don't open the door to this room again. Go!" Sue pointed to the door as she delivered these sentiments in a quiet voice.

"What if I refuse to go?" taunted George.

"Then the police will do it for you," said Sue, unperturbed and with that George stumped out of the room mumbling to himself as he went. The door closed and Sue wept silently into the eiderdown.

Chapter 8
Elizabeth Sweeney

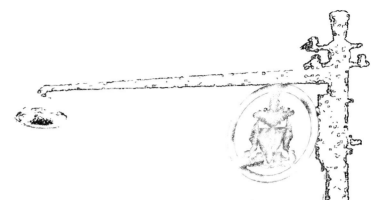

Nell had heard about Sue Taylor's ectopic pregnancy at the Primary Health Care Team meeting and thought she would pop in to see her this morning when she was in that neck of the woods.

That was a sad thing to happen, Nell thought as she walked along Nithsdale Road. Women often die with an ectopic pregnancy, due to delay in its diagnosis. They usually accredited the pain to a gastric upset, something that was too spicy, or that they had eaten too much.

Sue's door was ajar when Nell got to the house.

She shouted in, "Hello Sue, its Sister Dickson, I thought that I would pop in and see you today, as I heard that you were home from hospital."

"In you come, Sister, I'm through in the living room, come away through," Sue replied cheerily.

Nell was surprised to see Sue looking as spry, as she had heard that it was touch and go for a few hours after her surgery.

"I'm pleased to see you on your feet," said Nell earnestly, "and I am so, so sorry for your loss."

Sue pursed her lips and nodded repeatedly in response, but did not try to speak for a few moments. Then she said, "That blood they gave me must have been donated by a big strapping highland policeman, because I'm feeling as good as new." Then she laughed, "I'm exaggerating a bit but I'm really feeling heaps better now."

There was some Beatles music in the background from upstairs and Nell asked, "Is Christine off school today?" as she tilted her head in the direction of the music.

"Yes I kept her off. In actual fact, I think she'll need some counseling. Everything that's happened has been overwhelming. It's all been too traumatic for her. Sister, would you have a wee chat with Christine?"

"Yes, I'll be glad to do that Sue," replied Nell, "although I do think that you're so right thinking of professional help, if she doesn't come through this."

"She was so strong and took control when I collapsed with the pain," said Sue. "I thought that she was taking everything in her stride."

"Yes, the doctor told me how remarkable she was. Good for her, I think that she takes after her mother there!" replied Nell.

"She did well and saved my life in doing so…but yesterday I found her in a flood of tears, just sobbing she was."

"I can see why you kept her off school. She's still in an emotional state," Nell acknowledged.

"Christine firmly believes that because she was angry at me having the baby, she caused me to lose it, and through that, I found out that George was messing about again and I told him to pack up and leave permanently," explained Sue.

"Poor girl, she thinks that it is all her fault—losing the baby and her Dad," empathized Nell, then added; "I didn't know that George had gone for good."

"Well Sister, I have lost count of the number of new beginnings I have given him over the years and his old affair is new again. So I just took the bull by the horns so to speak," Sue smiled a wry smile, "and do y'know that I feel as if a huge weight's been lifted off me. I didn't realize that he was pulling me down so much with worry."

"Well you know yourself how you feel about things," said Nell. "It's great that you feel less of a burden now."

"Y'know, my granny, who left me this house, put in her will that George Taylor must never hold title deeds…even if I died first the house would be put into trust for the girls and any other offspring…she was a good judge of character."

"She must have been some Lady, in her day," smiled Nell.

"She was, and I think of her often, especially over the past few days. I remember the first time I thought George was unfaithful to me. I was so depressed that I felt like killing myself. In tears, I phoned my granny and told her so…she nearly exploded!

She shouted down the phone, 'Lassie, with George Taylor you contemplate murder, never suicide!' She made me laugh—she had such a quick wit!"

"How are you really coping with losing the pregnancy Sue?"

"I'm sad about losing the baby," Sue bit her lip and paused for a long moment, "but I'm reevaluating my life at the moment. George's mother and sister are going to move in to the big house with me and I am going to rent out the apartment that is a four room and kitchen. That will give me a bit of extra income.

With George's mother living here, it is a constant for the girls and they just love her and it will be less of an upset for his sister. I have always got on well with Lisa, George's mother; we have always been kindred spirits. George takes after his father in the affairs department, y'know. Lisa had a life of it and was left with a handicapped daughter. She knows what I have been putting up with for years. We will see how these new arrangements work out."

"You've certainly been doing a bit of planning, that's great," encouraged Nell.

"Well, I went to see the family lawyer and we looked at all my options. I would like to keep working if I can, as I enjoy the challenges it brings and it provides a social outlet too. I have true friends there," said Sue.

"It will be good for you to pick up the reins again when you are ready," said Nell.

"If you know of any one who is looking for a place to rent let me know."

"Oh! Now I may know of just the person," said Nell thinking instantly of Isa Carmichael.

Nell was amazed that Sue had radically changed a few things in her life. She had come to terms with these shattering life events. The impact of the changes, however, she would feel, and grapple with, for a long time to come. Sue was protecting her girls and that was her main focus. Nell marveled at Sue's respect for and her kindness towards her mother-in-law and handicapped sister-in-law.

Sue focused back on Christine, as another new record was played upstairs. "The other thing that has Christine totally confused is Jenny's circumstances. I really do not know what is happening on that front. Jenny did come in to see me when I was in the Samaritan, but I didn't like to pry, as she was there as a patient too. Whatever she was going through couldn't have been pleasant for the poor girl. I did tell her that my door would always be open for her and there's always a bed for her too."

"That is very kind of you Sue. Jenny is scarce in the real friend department you know," said Nell fighting back a tear. Sue worrying about Jenny, when she has so much to cope with herself, made Nell gulp.

"Oh I mean it Sister; I'm not just saying it y'know, Jenny has been a good friend to Christine. They chatted together when Christine came to visit me in the Samaritan and Jenny told her that she would tell everything one day when it didn't hurt so much. They plan to do their nursing training together; they have had that joint plan a few years now; they are really good friends."

"Well all I know is that there has definitely been abuse, just as you thought," said Nell. "You did the right thing in telling me about Jenny and we know that she is safe at present. There will be a court case and that's as far as I know. I don't know where Jenny was going when she left the Samaritan. I doubt if she will ever be back home again."

There was the noise of footsteps on the stairs, and then Christine appeared.

"Christine, this is Sister Dickson," said Sue as Christine came into the room, "I'll put the kettle on and Sister would like to explain a few things to you, OK?"

"I suppose," said Christine softly, her head hanging down and her mouth pursed to one side.

"Come and sit beside me if you like," said Nell, indicating to Christine as she took her hand in a warm handshake.

"I would like first to explain what an ectopic pregnancy is. Ask me any questions you want, there is no such thing as a silly question in my book," reassured Nell, smiling.

Christine smiled back, which lit up her face and put a little sparkle in her sad eyes. She had the good looks of her mother and father combined, and was already taller than her Mum. She was dressed in her school uniform, as she had tried to go to school that morning, but just could not stop crying. She wore a grey pleated school skirt, yellow shirt-blouse with the gold and navy school tie hanging loosely round her neck and a grey knitted cardigan. Her dark hair was scraped into a ponytail, but generous bangs and side wisps of wavy hair framed her pale face.

Nell proceeded to take a pad of paper from her case and drew the female reproductive organs on it. She began explaining the route that the fertilized ovum took on its way to the womb. Christine nodded and said the occasional "yes'" as she was familiar with this biology.

"So you see, there was no chance for this pregnancy to survive when the tube ruptured here," Nell put an X on the drawing. "Very occasionally the tube erodes slowly and the sac migrates into the abdominal cavity and the pregnancy survives as an abdominal pregnancy. I have only known about one of these in my time as a nurse and it was in Ireland…Belfast I think."

"So it wasn't anybody's fault then," stated Christine.

"That is right Christine, no one was to blame." Nell was going to add that it often happened after therapeutic abortions if there was infection, but she didn't, as Sue was listening to the explanation.

"Many women die from this, as they need surgical intervention right away," said Nell. Then she added, "If you had not been here for your Mum and not acted as quickly as you did, your Mum might not have made it."

Sue came over and hugged Christine. They both were crying and Nell was misty too and blew her nose hard, then said, "I'll pour the tea, OK?"

¤

It was 8:30 a.m. when Nell called in to see Isa Carmichael, who was looking so different since she had the baby. She was much slimmer and her face looked half the size it had been from that day she went into hospital. They exchanged hellos, then Nell asked, "Have you heard about your house yet Isa?"

"Nothing Sister, I think that they have forgotten me. I do hope that I hear soon, as I am beginning to hate this set up. Yesterday some kids here roughed up Sarah. They took her school hat and threw it into a puddle, then pushed her down. The wee soul skinned both her knees and the insides of her hands. She was really upset and came in crying sore," replied Isa leading the way through to the living room. "I'm trying my hardest to have a homey atmosphere here, but what's the use if the kids are afraid to go out?"

"I know of a place in Pollokshields that will be available soon," said Nell "I will give you the number and you can see if it meets your needs. Just mention my name."

"Thanks Sister, I am very much obliged."

"Now where's that wee cherub of yours?" asked Nell.

"Here he is!" said Isa, as she lifted baby Neil from the Moses basket and handed him to Nell.

"Well there wee man, you've grown a lot since I last saw you!" exclaimed Nell.

Nell and Isa spoke about the baby's weight and feeding and how Elizabeth was coping with her new brother. Nell was pleased to hear that the police had new evidence, which would show that Jake was not solely responsible for the fraudulent deal, so Isa was hoping for a lightened sentence when his appeal was held next month.

"Will you take a cup of tea Sister?" asked Isa.

"Thanks Isa, but I have to get on my way today. I just wanted to give you Sue Taylor's phone number without delay." Nell put Neil back in his Moses basket and wrote the number down for Isa.

"Thanks for this and for coming in to see us. Isn't it nice to see the Sister again, Elizabeth?" Elizabeth was clinging to her mother's skirt like a limpet and playing shy with Nell.

"Cheerio for now and I hope things work out for you house wise, Isa."

With that, Nell was on her way walking toward Crown Street to do some return visits for a neighbouring midwife who was stuck out at a confinement. She was going into a close in Crown Street when, out of the corner of her eye, she saw a wee boy on the other side of the street coming out of a close mouth. He was obviously going to school with his brown leather school bag high on his back and a large muffler tied in a smooth flap under his chin. Nell thought there was something odd in his behavior.

There was a go-chair parked at the close-mouth, with a large baby strapped into it. The baby, who looked to be about ten months old, was sitting up chewing on a toy. Nell stood in the shadows and watched the boy hesitate beside the baby. The boy looked distinctively suspicious. What was the wee twerp up to? He looked both ways and then looked back into the close then, in a flash, he took something from the baby and put it in his mouth. He stood there stooping and as he looked round, Nell saw that it was a dummy tit that was pinned onto the baby's coat. Here was the boy sucking hard on the dummy, having a wee fix before he went to school! He then left the baby and carried on his way to his place of learning!

Nell chuckled to herself the rest of the day. Growing up was hard. She found herself telling her next patient about what she had seen and they both laughed and Mary said, "Awe the shame."

Mary Murphy had been constipated. It was three days since the baby had been born and no bowel movement for Mary. The midwife that visited yesterday told her to get some glycerin suppositories from the chemist shop and take two that night. If the desired result did not happen she had to take another two this morning. Nell arrived to see her and was told the tale of the suppositories.

"And have your bowels moved yet Mary?" asked Nell directly.

"Whit bowls Sister?" said Mary not quite comprehending.

"Did you have a good shite yet?" said Nell using the Glasgow term for fecal matter and thus avoiding any further euphemisms or misunderstandings.

"Naw Sister that's the poablim ye see, Ah hivni' goan since Friday," Mary said, back on track, "an Aah took two o' they supposed thingies and nothing his come, an' they wur awful things tae swallae!"

"Well," said Nell, "that will keep your inside lubricated for a wee while, but I'll show you the best way to use them. Just lie on the bed Mary, roll over and pull up your knees a little."

Nell flipped on a finger cot and inserted two suppositories into Mary's rectum. "Now just lie there for about twenty minutes and see if that makes a difference."

"Help ma' kiltie!" said Mary, "Is that whit yi hid tae dae wi' them things. That wis the first time Ah hid ever saw them," said Mary.

"Well how were you to know unless it was explained to you," said Nell kindly. "I had never seen them either till I started nursing. In our house, if there was a problem in that department it was a spoonful of Syrup of Figs or Castor Oil. In fact, many families had a weekly doze whether they needed it or not!" They both laughed.

"I'll be the talk o' the Steamie if this gets oot," chuckled Mary.

They both laughed louder, then Mary had to dash to the loo. It was wonderful, the way that the Glasgow folk could laugh at themselves. Nell told Mary about her own sister May who had been on holiday in Venice when she was rushed to hospital in the ambulance Gondola with severe abdominal pain. They thought that it was appendicitis.

All the nurses were Nuns and none of them spoke English. May did not speak any Italian, except for a few travelers' phrases. She was feeling really ill and was lying with the screens round her when this Nun appeared with a silver tray covered with a snow white starched linen drape. May thought that she was about to get the Last Rites' of the Catholic Church. She desperately called out to the Nun, "Non Catholique, Non Catholique," but the Nun did not alter her approach. She pulled the bedclothes off May, rolled her on her left side and inserted two rectal suppositories! Then she was gone as swiftly as she had appeared.

May felt really stupid! Instructions had to be crystal clear. There was no telling how things were interpreted and what the results would be. Nell remembered one case where what she had said was completely misunderstood. It was early spring. She remembered that because the birds were singing as she left the Kaur's house about 6:30 in the morning. She had been there all night from about seven o'clock the previous evening. It had been a long night.

This was Surjeet Kaur's first baby. Surjeet was a sweet girl from Goa and had come on her own to Glasgow for an arranged marriage. She was trying hard to learn English. She had only been in Britain for eighteen months and lived with her husband, his parents and young brother-in-law, who was still at school.

Granny Kaur was delighted, as this was her first Grandson. They lived in Abbotsford Place but owned the whole flat, which was spacious and bright. The house was sparkling clean and granny Kaur, every time she saw Nell, would say, "Tea?" There were only so many cups of tea one could drink.

The baby suckled at the breast, but there was nothing there. He was howling and the mother and granny would not put him back to the breast. They wanted to give the baby a bottle. Many of the Indian and Pakistani women would breastfeed their babies successfully from the seventh day after birth. It was also the practice in Glasgow at that time to feed the baby boiled water first.

Not having any powdered milk with her, and the fact that it was a Sunday morning and the shops were all closed, Nell wrote out the instructions of how to modify cow's milk for baby use. Nell knew that there was a Chemist open from 2–4 p.m. and she would also bring some free samples with her later that day. She went over the instructions many times and even spoke to the young brother-in-law about it. All seemed clear about how to modify the cow's milk for baby. Nell returned about 11 a.m. and found the baby ravenous, sucking the satin binding on the blanket as Granny Kaur shook him up and down in a desperate effort to comfort her grandson.

"Did you not give the baby any cow's milk?" Nell asked.

"No Sister, my husband he say we no room to keep a cow!" explained Surjeet in a serious tone. Nell wondered what the scene would have been if they did have room!

She had heard from another midwife that one young immigrant mum had bought a big bottle of Milk of Magnesia for her new baby. All she recognized was the word "milk" and thought that it must be good for the baby. Cow's milk or doorstep milk was the bottled milk available; either Tuberculin Tested (TT) milk from TT herds or pasteurized milk, which had undergone heat treatment to kill the bovine tuberculosis bacilli.

The other headache for the Green Ladies, both the midwives and the health visitors, was the problem of the "extra scoop". Mothers had somehow been brain washed that if an extra scoop of powered milk went into the night bottle feed, it would satisfy the baby more and result in a longer sleep. This was totally wrong and caused dehydration and over a long period of time posed the risk of permanent kidney damage.

Nell encouraged breast feeding, as all the midwives did, but bottle feeding was in Vogue: National Dried Milk was produced by the government and available at the health clinics at a lower cost than the brand names. All the dried milk powders came in half cream and full cream strengths. Much time was taken to educate new mothers on how to make up a bottle, how to sterilize the bottles and when to gradually switch to full cream!

There was also tinned Carnation evaporated milk or another brand of evaporated milk, both of which had instructions written on the side in minute lettering. These instructions were always being misread and the midwives spent a lot of time individualizing bottle-feeding teaching for new mothers.

Nell went further down Crown Street to do another visit. This was a notorious family. Elizabeth Sweeney, the matriarch, ruled with a rod of Iron. There were eleven children in the family; "his, mine an' oors," Elisabeth had once told Nell.

Elizabeth was a large woman of five feet nine in height and twenty stones in non-pregnant weight. She had a flushed face and auburn wiry, frizzy, curly hair that she wore in a short style created by her own pinking shears! Her hair looked like "Oor Wullie's" hair, in technicolour. Her eyes were a piercing sky blue and when she looked directly at you, you could almost feel her gaze piercing your skin. Her bosom was large, but in proportion to the rest of her bulk. She was usually dressed in a large floral print drindle skirt with a flounce of about eight inches at the bottom. This allowed her to sit with her legs wide apart and be adequately covered. She always wore blouses with the modesty vest insert to shield the cleavage. The modesty vest was usual apparel for the older generation but fashion, friend or foe did not argue with Elizabeth Sweeney. Her ankles were solidly chunky and adequately planted in a pair of black velvet pumps, were known as ballerina pumps. Stockings were absent; she wore none.

Upon entering the old style kitchen, it was dark. Nell wondered sometimes if keeping the place dark was to confuse the head count. Once you were there for a while, and your eyes accommodated to the darkness, forms of people emerged out of the background. The coal-fired range was the centerpiece of the room. It was gleaming, as it had been freshly black leaded by one of the girls; it was unclear if the girl was "his, mine or oors."

There were two pulleys running the full length of the room, each with three rungs, and both laden with washing. Many items were hanging full length from them. Nell thought it must be some weight to hoist one of these pulleys when full of wet clothes. Running the same direction as the pulleys stood cabinets on the opposite wall from the range. There were two low storage cupboards and a coal bunker, all of which provided a work surface on top. The coal bunker lid was hinged to allow the coal man to deliver the coal. It also had a flap at the front for easy access to the coal. The window was at one end of the room and the bed recess, complete with bed, at the other end of the room. The curtains at the window matched the curtains round the bed recess and each pair had a top frill. They were beige in colour with a large red rose pattern, which was almost luminous in the dark kitchen.

The kitchen was never empty. The kettle was never off the boil. The Glasgow "patter" never ceased. Elizabeth would not let any one call her Lizzy or Beth; her mother was called Lizzy and her granny had been called Beth. Elizabeth ran a catalogue account for General Stores; she took delivery of the catalogues. People came to her kitchen to choose their desired merchandise, which she sent for, and they brought the money to her each week. The company, in turn, paid Elizabeth 10% commission. She liked to see fair play and stood no nonsense from any one! Elizabeth did not have trouble in collecting the weekly remittances. It was commonly desirable to be listed in her good books.

Nell knocked on the door, which immediately swung open.

"It's the Sister, can I come in Elizabeth?" Nell called out into a darkish hallway.

"Aye, in ye come, hen, am in ra' kitchen," came the reply.

"How are you doing, Elizabeth?" asked Nell as she got her breath back after climbing the stairs.

"Fair to middlin' hen, quite a lot o' they efter pains and ah huv decided tae pit the wean on the national dried milk, jist like the last three," decreed Elizabeth and there would be no argument there.

"Good. I know that you will add enough sugar and the right amount of boiled water to make it safe for him," reminded Nell in a non-threatening way.

The "him" was a 12 lb, 4 oz cherub. He had a shock of black hair and looked like the baby of the Michelin X Man. He really looked like the baby of a diabetic mother.

"Is he demanding to be fed every three hours or there abouts?" asked Nell.

"Aye, but he only takes three oonces at a time," replied Elizabeth.

"Yes, he only has a baby sized stomach and he will probably lose weight first, before he starts putting some on. Did the doctor say that he would like you to have a glucose tolerance test done?"

"Aye," said Elizabeth, "but I don't think I'll bother wi' that hen."

Nell left the matter there, as Elizabeth's own doctor and midwife would sort that one out. They would probably arrange for her to have the test done at home.

Nell knew Elizabeth suffered from agoraphobia and had not been over the door in two years; not since the funeral of her ten year old son Sam. Sam had been knocked down by a Lorry in Crown Street, not far from his home. He had been playing football in a vacant lot and the ball rolled onto the road and he followed it. He was the first of the "oor" children.

Elizabeth did not have a recent photograph of Sam, so the coroner took one for her. She had the photograph framed. It had pride of place on the mantelpiece. The photograph looked odd; the eyes were staring and were expressionless, but it was better than not having a photograph of her boy. She had a little vase beside the photograph and always had a single fresh flower in it or some forget-me-nots when she could get them.

Elizabeth did not go out into the world; the world came to her. People trickled in from morning till night, bringing their stories and gossip with them. The kitchen was to the back of the house and in the summer Elizabeth would take a cushion through to the parlour at the front of the house, open one of the sash windows and place the cushion on the window sill. Then she would place a chair in front of it and proceed to look out of the window and lean on the cushion. This was a custom in the Glasgow tenements and was termed "hingin oot the windae." It was amazing what neighbourhood goings-on were noted from a wee "hing out the windae!"

Elizabeth did not venture out and refused all help in that department. That was one reason that she had piled on the body fat. When Nell was checking Elizabeth's abdomen, she found a biro pen in the fat folds, Nell put the pen on the table.

"Oh thanks hen…" Elizabeth had said "…Ah loast that a couple o' days ago, ah wondered where it hid went".

When her children would act up she would yell at them, "Wait till yer faither gets hame, he'll sort ye oot."

Nell always thought that Ed Sweeney was a giant of a man matching Elizabeth in size, but he was a wee thin man of five feet four under his "bunnet", which seemed to be permanently attached to his head. They looked like the comic characters "Andy Cap and Florrie"—large wife and wee husband. It reminded Nell of her biology teacher talking about the ovum and the sperm; female is large and sessile, and the male is small and mobile. Ed was mobile all right; he was a hard worker and was a docker at the Govan docks. He made good money and he always seemed to have a few of the fringe benefits; when a case loads of goods "fell aff a lorry". Elizabeth could sell anything in her own domain as the neighbourhood filtered through her kitchen.

Nell had commented, "What a lovely lamp," while looking at a painted globular base and matching painted lampshade.

"Aye that's only wan an' a penny a week so it is, an that picture up there is only two an' tanner a week," said Elizabeth.

Nell looked at the picture of a large elephant in an African Jungle scene. It did seem a trifle out of place in a kitchen in Gorbals, but it did make an artistic statement for "two an' a tanner a week". The weekly payment allowed the neighbourhood women to buy a few niceties for their home as long as it did not get the better of them. What Elizabeth did not say was the number of weeks it took to pay the lamp or the picture off completely—probably at least twenty or thirty weeks!

The deprivation cycle was always at work. Women, being poor and deprived of any luxury, would splurge out on something that they did not really need and in the end, made them the poorer. At Christmas, this was evident. They would buy their children the most expensive toys and put themselves in deep debt to the likes of General Stores. The glow and magic of Christmas morning would soon fade, the toy would break and the harsh reality of paying a pound a week to Elizabeth Sweeney for the next ten months would seem endless. Elizabeth Sweeney had an open ear for all and if the elephant on her wall could talk, what stories it could tell!

Nell finished the visit and the people who had left the room for Nell to complete her visit with Elizabeth in private, filed back into the room. Nell then buttoned her green double-breasted coat, slipped the green belt through the green bakelite buckle and tugged to tighten it. She lifted her case and bade farewell to the assembled shoppers.

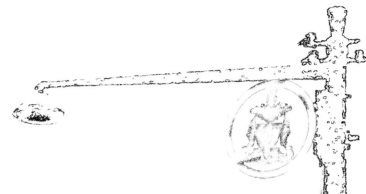

Chapter 9
George Taylor

George Taylor was absolutely stunned! He sat at the wheel of his car and stared at the windscreen. Had it really happened? Had Sue really told him to go? It had hit him like a ton of bricks! It all happened so quickly and he packed his things in record time without a second thought. He could not say anything to the girls; he could not face them. He was too embarrassed when it came to them. They had so much insight into things that it unnerved him.

He'd better phone Patsy and tell her that her wish had come true. George was excited! He felt free and happy. Should he surprise Patsy and brighten up her dull evening with a visit from her lover boy, as he had told her he couldn't see her tonight? She had been so distraught about it when they had met for a quick lunch. The car engine roared as it drove out of the driveway, scattering the red sandstone chips on its way, and headed for Glasgow's town center.

At that moment Patsy was at home looking over Jason Adams' art portfolio. Jason was a student art teacher who was allocated to Patsy's department for a four-week practical experience and he was no doubt going to get just that and more from Patsy, by the way she was sizing him up. Adam was keen to show off his portfolio.

Pasty invited him to her place straight from school. She had been eyeing him up all afternoon. Jason was medium height and had a receding hairline that made him look older than his 22 years. He was very muscular and proud of it.

Patsy was commenting on one of his paintings, "I just love the subtle hues here with the light falling over the trees."

He came up behind her, as she had hoped he would, to see what she was pointing out and his breath fell on her ear, neck and even down the cleavage of her low cut blouse. His nearness evoked a heavy scent of musk in her nostrils and she leaned back onto him heaving her breasts with her next breath. Jason steadied her with his arms around her waist.

She wriggled into him, stroking his arms and said, "Well that feels really nice Jason Adams," and she let the painting float to the floor as her small thin frame squirmed round in his arms to look into his now flushed face.

She held his face in her hands and gently kissed him on the lips. He immediately returned the kiss in an ardent embrace, swaying her body back toward the couch. In a flash, they were deep in the couch cushions. He was kissing her with all the urgency of youth, his hands fondling her breasts and unbuttoning her low-necked blouse.

She reached under his sweater and was pleased to find only a vest, which she pulled out of his trousers and in one upward thrust his well-developed chest was naked. The vest covered sweater bundle flew away as their naked breasts touched. Heavy breathing turned to panting between kisses as they feverishly stripped the lower garments off each other; he kissed her naked body all over.

He sure knows all the erogenous areas, Patsy thought. He has done this before. She was now fully aroused and clung to his neck, her pelvis writhing under him. She moaned when she felt him thrust again and again as they made love fast and furiously. Their bodies stiffened together in climax and then slumped in release.

"That is some portfolio you have, Mr. Adams!"

"Thank you for taking the time to appreciate it, Miss Orr."

They rolled off the couch onto the floor laughing.

"Beep beep beep. Here is the six o'clock news for Wednesday…" the BBC radio announcer said.

"Crivens! Is that the time already," exclaimed Jason "I better rush to catch the bus. I have football practice at the fifty pitches at seven. Can I leave my portfolio here with you Patsy? I don't fancy carrying it all the way there and back. It may get damaged in the dressing rooms, they are so tight for space."

"Sure, I will bring it to school in the morning for you."

"Thanks, you are a doll."

Dressed, portfolio packed and carefully placed in the hallway, glass of juice downed, Jason was gone like a whirlwind and no doubt pleased that he had scored before the game.

Patsy cleaned up and was drinking a large mug of tea on the sexy couch, thinking of the impetuousness of the young. They think that they invented the sex act! She smiled with pleasure and took a big gulp of hot sweet tea. Suddenly, the piercing ring of the doorbell entered her musings.

"What has he left behind?" she said aloud.

She opened the door nonchalantly, expecting to see Jason and there stood eager eyed George, with his two suitcases in hand.

"Surprise surprise!" he exclaimed. "I'm here to stay, just as you wanted! I have left Sue and I'm all yours, Patsy my girl. You can close your mouth now doll."

Patsy could not take it all in. Twice she had been called "doll' in a short space of time! She took a double take. She did close her mouth, which was wide with astonishment.

"Am I not welcome?" asked George a wee bit miffed. "I feel a bit like the man who fell out the balloon, you know I'm not in it at all!"

His head tilted to the side, trying in vain to elicit a normal Patsy response that he was familiar with. "It's a surprise then?"

"George it's no surprise. It's a bloody shock! Of course you are more than welcome, come in, come away in."

George brought his luggage into the spacious hallway. He was really pleased that he had given Patsy a surprise.

"Been working?" asked George referring to the portfolio.

"No, it's not mine; I brought it home to have a closer look at it. Have you eaten yet?" she asked diverting his attention away from Jason's artwork.

"No, have you?" answered George.

"Not yet."

"Then let me take you out for a quick bite to celebrate. OK?" suggested George.

"Sure that will be great, and you can tell me all about the break up," Patsy said, glad for the time to recoup her cool.

"You look a bit flustered and tired Patsy," George commented.

"Oh I have had a busy day. We have had student teachers in this week and you know how exhausting they can be."

"I guess so," George replied. "Let me help you with your coat, Mrs. Taylor to be."

Patsy wasn't sure that she liked the sound of that, but she kissed him on the cheek anyway. He held the door open for her and she swanned through. She heard her mother's voice in her mind saying, "Be careful what you wish for girl, you might just get it!" They left for a celebration dinner with minds on somewhat different planes.

¤

Saturday dawned and the phone rang.

"Jenny! I'm so pleased to hear your voice," said Christine into the receiver.

"How are you?" There was a pause and then, "See you soon then, that's great! I'll walk up towards the station." Christine put the receiver down and ran to find her mother. "Mum, Jenny is on her way here. I said I would walk towards the station to meet her."

"That's nice, I hope she can stay for dinner," said Sue. "Christine, I need to talk to you about Jenny before she comes. I need to prepare you so that you won't get too big a shock should Jenny tell you what she has been through."

"OK Mum."

"I will try to be really clear. Her father and her brother have sexually abused Jenny. That means that they have raped her many times. They told her that she would ruin the family if she told anyone. Do you know what rape is?"

"Yes and no, Mum. I know it's not what Fiona said that time in the car, is it?" she smiled.

"No it isn't," said Sue. Christine was recalling a time when she and Fiona (who was only seven at the time) were in the back of the car. They were stopped at traffic lights and Christine read the news headlines on newspaper boards, "GIRL RAPED". She immediately asked Sue what raped meant and there was silence as Sue searched for the best way to explain this with Fiona present. The silence was broken by Fiona's cheery voice, "You know, you rake up the leaves? So, the girl was raked!" Sue let it pass at that!

"It means that, against her will, she was held down and forced to have sexual intercourse," explained Sue.

"Oh! Mum that is awful!" exclaimed Christine with a look of horror on her face. "How could she bear it? That was really beastly!" she continued with a screwed up look of disgust on her face. "Ooo! That's disgusting! Thanks for getting it stopped!" cried Christine and she threw her arms round her mother.

"Don't pry into Jenny's affairs, Christine. She is working through a lot of grief just now. She will tell you in time, perhaps a little bit at a time."

"OK Mum, I won't ask anything. I better run now," and she was off out the door.

Sue thought it was so good to see Christine looking forward to meeting her friend again.

Jenny arrived and the girls had a good time playing their latest records and catching up on school gossip. Jenny shared a few things with Christine. She told her she was staying with foster parents in Newlands and it was an easy train ride to Pollokshields to see Christine. She and one brother were together and her father and other brother were serving prison sentences. The third brother was still in the family home. Jenny did not say much more than giving these living arrangements, but she knew that Christine had an understanding of what had happened. Jenny knew that Christine felt some loss too, as her father was living with his girlfriend.

Christine asked Jenny if she would like to meet the girl next door. The Carmichaels had moved in a few weeks ago. She told her all about the twins.

"Tom is always away at the weekends, but I will introduce you to Sarah and her wee sister Emma who has chummed up with Fiona. They cycle everywhere together."

Jenny said, "Don't say about me being in foster care."

"Please don't worry about that, I would never do anything to hurt you, you will always be my best friend, Jenny." The two girls hugged and went off chatting, to see the Carmichaels.

Sarah Carmichael was painting a picture with watercolours when they arrived. She was so pleased to see them, and so was Isa, who immediately said, "I'll bring you through some lemonade and biscuits girls."

The threesome talked about their three different schools—Bellahouston Academy, Shawlands Academy, and Laurelbank School for Girls. There seemed to be the same class of "bitches" in each school and they laughed about it. Then they decided to go for a walk to Bellahouston Park and check out the tennis schedule for the next Saturday.

Isa had a tear in her eye as she watched them go down the path chatting incessantly. It had been a long time since Sarah had had some company her own age at the weekends. Isa dialed the number, "Fancy a wee cup o'char Sue?"

The two women sat in Isa's kitchen blathering over a cup of tea and Isa's newly baked hot treacle scones with lashings of butter. Their hearts were bountiful because their daughters had a little bit of normalcy in their young troubled lives.

Sue then said, "Jenny is staying for dinner so why don't I take Elizabeth and baby David and the girls for dinner too. Fiona just loves Elizabeth and the baby and so do I. You can take a break, have a night out."

"Will it not be too much trouble?" asked Isa.

"Not at all," reassured Sue. "George's mother and sister love to have a crowd, too. Lisa is a good help and Sammy loves to play with Elizabeth. So you do what ever you want."

Baby David Carmichael was outnumbered that night with all these women fussing over him, as his Dad, Jake, lay in his prison cell trying to figure out who set him up to be the fall guy.

¤

"Hello Sister, nice to see you," said Geoff, as Nell entered the Easy Eats café. "How's it goin?"

"Oh fine, I'm meeting the student here this morning Geoff. I'll have a cup of coffee and a Paris bun please," replied Nell.

"Coming right up Sister," said Geoff. "A coffee for the Sister, please May, an'a fresh Paris bun."

"Good morning Sister, here's your coffee then," greeted May as she served Nell.

"How are you May?" asked Nell.

"Fair to middlin' Sister. The weans goat a bad coaff an A've been up hoaff the night," replied a very tired looking May.

"Did you take him to see the doctor May?" asked Nell.

"Naw, no yit."

"See if you can get in today as there is a bad flu about," advised Nell.

"Aye Sister I'll dae jist that."

The door swung open and into the Café came a bustling Jane Andrews, the student midwife. She was from sunny Jamaica and had a jovial nature to match.

"Hello Sister!" she said brightly, "I am Jane Andrews, am I late?"

"Pleased to meet you Jane, I'm Sister Dickson. No you're not late, please sit down. Will you have a cup of coffee and something to eat, on me."

"Thanks sister, yes I would love coffee and an egg roll. I just love these Scottish morning rolls. I did not take the time to have breakfast, in case I missed that bus."

"We have plenty of time and I will tell you our plan for today. That is, unless someone goes into labour."

They had a busy morning, but Jane was a very competent nurse. Nell found out that she had a child in Jamaica.

"Well Sister, you are more marriageable if you have had one child. It proves that you are not barren. My mother looks after him and I will look after her in turn."

In one house, when Jane was just finishing bathing the baby and the big brother of four was studying her, Nell knew by the intent look on his face that a question of profound importance was about to issue forth from his wee mouth. Nell tried to distract him, but to no avail.

"Does that black not come off when you wash your hands?" the big brother asked Jane.

"No it doesn't," replied Jane, unperturbed. "Come and I'll show you," and she lifted the baby bath to empty it. The big brother followed her to the sink and they both washed their hands and made bubbles. He inspected her hands back and front.

"My skin is black because I came from a very hot country. I have a little boy your size in that country and he has black skin too, and he likes fire trucks, just like you."

The next few mornings the big brother was waiting for Jane at the window and ran to greet her as soon as the doorbell rang.

Nell enjoyed Jane Andrew's company. She had a wonderful optimistic outlook on life. The time passed quickly.

One mother they visited insisted on putting extra scoops of dried baby milk power into the nighttime bottle-feed. There was a big push on to stop women from doing that, as research showed that permanent kidney damage could result. Nell had spent so much time with the mother and still she kept doing it.

When they got out of the house Nell turned to Jane and said, "You tell them till you are blue in the face but it does not seem to make any difference."

Jane's black face burst out laughing, Nell did too. "Sorry Jane, its just another Glasgow expression."

"Don't be, it's your usual form of speech, so don't change for me. It just struck me as funny that I would end up with a black and blue face!"

They were laughing together as they walked along the road when they heard a woman shouting, "Sister, Sister, can you come please?"

They both turned and saw a woman waving frantically to them from a third floor tenement building. They hurried up the flights of stairs and through the open door to find a man in his seventies in respiratory distress. He was a thin man and he was gasping for breath. He had a blue circle round his mouth and was making a great effort on inspiration. There were beads of sweat on his forehead. Nell took his pulse and respiration rate; both were elevated. She had a few words with his wife and had a look at the medications he was on.

"We have to get you into hospital, Dougie. They will be able to clear this fluid that is causing the breathlessness. I will give you this Amyl Nitrate pill for under your tongue. I know you don't have your heart pain just now, but it will relieve your bronchospasm."

Nell wrote a message for Jane to phone the doctor's surgery from the Café. "I will stay with you till the ambulance comes," Nell reassured Dougie.

The wife, Anne, said that Dougie had been vomiting and hadn't taken his diuretic pill for a few days. Nell gave him his dose there and then.

"It will help a little, but they will be able to give you an injection of the diuretic for a more dramatic result when you get to the hospital," Nell explained.

"Thanks Sister," said Dougie's wife. "I didnae want tae leave him to phone the doctor and its ma' neebours day for the steamie, so she hus been away since early."

"Not to worry," said Nell. "I'm pleased to help. Can you open that window a bit more and give him some fresher air?"

She gently sponged Dougie's hands and face and got him to relax and do some abdominal breathing. This relaxed him a bit, but his lips remained blue.

The ambulance came quickly and Dougie and Anne went off to the Victoria Infirmary. As they helped Anne into the ambulance she was thanking Jane and Nell profusely.

"What can you do?" Nell discussed with Jane. "You must lend a hand in a case like that. We are not supposed to do general cases, but I don't think that he was infectious, just in heart failure. How about a bite of lunch at the Easy Eats Café and we will organize the afternoon's visits?"

Off they trotted along Cumberland Street, chatting about the high rate of respiratory problems in the inner city. Nell related the case of the family near her who succumbed to tuberculosis, and three of the teenage children and the mother died. This stuck in Nell's mind, although she was just a child, as they were strikingly handsome boys with jet black curly hair and the sister had long, shiny black, pleats of her hair right down her back that she could sit on. Nell decided then to be a scientist and find a cure for TB. There was a cure before she grew up so, she was then free to be a nurse!

¤

In her general training, Nell spent time working in the two TB wards in the Southern General Hospital—ward number seven and eight to be precise. She remembered these wards well because this is where she was taught to do Z-tract injections and the importance of strict barrier nursing.

She remembered that some of the patients looked well and did not believe that they had to take the deplorable tablets. Pas and Inah were the medications. Nell always thought that they sounded like a biblical couple! It took time to heal from tuberculosis. Nell used to give out the bottles of Stout to the men twice a week. The doctor believed that it helped their appetite. Nell celebrated her twenty-first birthday on this ward on night shift. The men were younger and were good fun. It was not fun for them to be away from home and be forced to rest, away from their active lives.

There had been a mass chest x-ray screening program throughout Britain and this caught early cases of tuberculosis that were then treated. This, with strict penalties for spitting in public places, brought tuberculosis under control. Nell remembered, as a child, learning to spell "spitting" from such a poster:

"Spitting Strictly Prohibited." She also could spell "strictly", but "prohibited" eluded her for some time to come. She thought it was some sort of "bite". The power of the printed word! Such posters were usually endorsed with "By Order". It seemed to Nell that God had made the poster, so it better be obeyed.

¤

"Hello Bridget," chorused Jenny, Christine, and Sarah as they reached the tennis courts at Bellahouston Park. Bridget was a girl who Christine had met playing tennis. Bridget went to Saint Gerrard's School, and Christine and Jenny had played them at Hockey in the inter-school matches. They had met her the previous Saturday and arranged to play tennis today. Bridget was pleased to play with them, as she did not see any of her schoolmates out of school because she lived a distance away.

Her parents were older. She was a "change of life baby" and all her brothers and sisters were married. She had eleven nieces and nephews and two of them were older than she was. Bridget was a lovely girl with thick auburn hair, which she wore in long ringlets. When she was out of sight of her mother she tied it back behind her neck with a pony tail elastic

The foursome played well together and arranged to go out in the evening to the Mosspark Picture House, to the first house showing of the picture. There was an Elvis film on that night. Afterwards they could walk along as far as the Bungalow Café and have a hot orange drink and a chocolate bar. This was living it up! And they would all be home by nine.

The girls' friendships deepened. They chatted, they laughed, they were serious about issues, they played tennis, they socialized, and in this way they helped each other along the troublesome adolescent path.

Nell's thoughts were very much with Jenny. She wished there were a cure for the social diseases that inflicted on the young girls and women she cared for. Nell was pleased to hear from Sue that Jenny was enjoying some normality, good times with good friends, and that she and Christine had continued a close friendship.

Jenny needs a good friend more than anyone, Nell thought.

Nell and Jane continued along Cumberland Street, case in hand, chatting as they went about the world of midwifery.

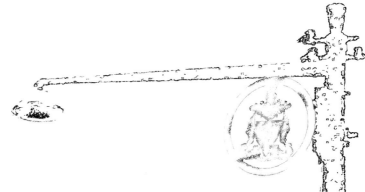

Chapter 10
Tess Arnott

"Sister, there is a call for a midwife to go to a house at Gorbals Cross." The voice on the phone was unclear. "Sounds as if there is a post partum hemorrhage on the go!"

"I'll go straight away," replied Nell.

"I have sent the message for the flying squad, but I thought if you get a taxi from the southside, you may get there first because it's rush hour."

Miss MacGreggor's voice was clearer now. Nell could always hear her voice repeating over in her mind, when the phone call was over.

The taxi arrived at record speed and the evening rush hour was just starting. The driver knew Glasgow well and ducked out and in the traffic, up and down side streets to avoid traffic lights. When it was an emergency they did their best to make time. Relating this would brighten up the taxi driver's dinner table conversation with his family that night. "I took a Green Lady on an emergency trip!"

When they got to the close, the police and the fire brigade were already there. Nell rushed up the stairs to the first floor. There was a fireman standing in an open doorway.

"This way Sister," he said as he beckoned her in. "Over there, the room to the right."

Nell walked in and the smell of booze could have knocked her down. There were wine bottles rolling about the floor. There in the bed recess bed, was the new mother.

Tess Arnott was slumped against the headboard of the bed,

her white floral nighty stained red. The bedclothes were heavily stained red with something, but it wasn't blood. There was not the peculiar stank odour of blood. Nell's first glance told her this was wine stains, not blood stains! A quick examination of the intoxicated woman and Nell called to the fireman outside the door. "Please contact the flying squad and cancel them…they are not needed here. OK?"

"OK Sister…will do…"

A few moments later came this reply, "too late, Sister, they're on their way."

"Thanks, can you tell them, as soon as they arrive, not to unpack their gear as there is no emergency here?" Nell called back to the fireman.

"Okey-dokey," came the prompt reply.

The baby was sleeping soundly, even though there were two persistent flies running all over the upturned rosy cheek. Flies swarmed about; over the Moses Basket, over the bedclothes, and over the sink area. The place was filthy and was in need of a good scrub. Nell lifted the baby and quickly washed her wee face clean of the dried in posseted milk that was attracting the flies.

Tommy Arnott, the man of the house, explained to Nell, through his drunken state, "Ye see hen, Ah hud goat ma' broo money and thoat that we wid celebrate the baby, ye ken, wet the wean's heed an' awe that. But hur, the big fool, goat stotious," he turned his head to the side and put a shaky back-of-his-hand to the side-of-his-red-nose and said in a loud stage whisper. "She could never hold her liquor anyway!"

The spray from the whisper spouted four feet in front of him. "And then we saw the blood oan the sheets an' she thought she wis bleedin' to death! She panicked! Ah wis scared, Ah didnae want tae lose her, ye ken, no jist yet anyway," he gave a wink, and a couple of nods of his head and continued. "So Ah yelled oot the windae an' goat a wee man tae phone fur help. Ah didnae know jist at that time wee Effie, up the stairs…" His eyes were blinking and his mouth was gaping, with his bottom lip quavering. He was trying to stay in the vicinity of the top lip, as he looked upwards to the ceiling into a clothes laden pulley, "…wis burnin' her toast, and the fat frae last night's sausages coat fire in the grill pan. She hid opened her windae tae let the smoke belch oot an' when the wee man, that wis gonnae phone fur me, looked up he thought that the place was burnin doon an he phoned the fire brigade an' that's hoo it aw sterted."

Amid all the confusion, and despite his mouth feverishly trying to locate its original home in the middle of his face, but never quite reaching the precise spot, he was coherent enough to be understood; probably a past master of this craft.

The flying squad arrived ready to save the life of the woman bleeding to death and Nell gave the story.

"Thanks Sister, for telling us to leave the gear in the ambulance," said the young doctor, who quickly assessed the situation then continued. "The traffic was absolutely diabolical on the bridge. I couldn't believe it. We could have walked here quicker…and that's the truth."

"We definitely need another bridge," Nell said. "It is just a bottleneck from about 3 till 6 every week day on all the bridges."

A crowd of about a hundred had gathered in the street. A press photographer and reporter from the Evening Citizen newspaper came to get the story on the house fire and wanted to know if the entire family had perished! News traveled fast and rumours had a heyday.

Once the emergency vehicles left, one policeman and Nell were left with the problem of an intoxicated couple in charge if three children under the age of four, when a kind neighbour came to the rescue. Pam, the neighbour, had just arrived home from work and came in to see if she could help. She was dressed in a white overall and wore a white linen turban through which you could see the outline of a head full of hair curlers. Pam worked in a biscuit factory in Hillington. It was refreshing to see someone clean and fresh, even after a day's work. She took charge of the children, so Nell and the police could go. They would check up the next day. Pam knew that if the children were taken into care it would take ages to get them returned to their parents.

She said in their defense, "They're no a bad pair Sister, jist a bit daft and scatterbrained. They both love they weans ye know. They like to come into see me, the wee yins do; they know Ah aye hae chocolate biscuits. Ah buy the reject biscuits oan a Friday; ye know the wans missing a wee bit chocolate, an the weans think that it's great. I'll feed and bath them wi ma three and they can sleep in ma place the night. Ah don't stert work till 2 in the efternoon ra morra. It'll be as right as rain Sister, don't you worry yersel."

Nell smiled a smile of gratitude. There was Pam, a single mother of three, willing to lend a big hand in a time of need. A Glasgow neighbour is indeed a treasure beyond worth, thought Nell.

On the way home on the bus, Nell mused over the cost of that little escapade. There seemed to be no accountability for wasting public funds.

Everyone was pleased and relieved though, that it was not a matter of life and death. It could all be blamed on wee Effie burning her toast or the fact that she had had sausages for her tea the night before and did not clean out the dripping in the grill pan!

Strangely enough, Nell met the midwife for that area about a month later and she learned that Tess Arnott did have a post partum hemorrhage three weeks later and had to be rushed to hospital by the flying squad. The bleeding would have been caused by infection no doubt, thought Nell, as hygiene went out the window there, just like wee Effie's smoke! Tess did survive, but it was touch and go for a few days. Some happenings were strange and a sense of déjà vu existed!

¤

"Oh Sister I think I am going to die, I have a terrible sinking feeling."

The words chilled Nell to the marrow. It was 3:30 a.m. in a quiet Glasgow street and barely a soul stirring. It was almost surreal. She checked the patient's pulse and blood pressure and they were fine. The baby had been born about 20 minutes ago and all had been normal. The placenta was then delivered and appeared complete. Nell gave Madge Sorley an intramuscular injection to stimulate the uterus to contract, massaged the fundus of the uterus till it was as hard as a cricket ball. The perineum was intact so no stitches were required. She cleaned the perineal area, put a fresh pad on and rolled the confinement sheet and tarred paper away.

All this Nell did on automatic pilot, as Madge's words filled her consciousness. "Sister I think I'm going to die." This scared Nell to the core! She re-checked pulse, blood pressure, temperature, fundus and lochial flow, and checked her legs for ensuing phlebitis; all was as normal as pie! What was she missing? She sent Alf, Madge's husband, out to phone for the doctor to come. There was no indication that any thing was wrong but, "Sister I think I'm going to die," spooked her. She had heard stories about the premonitions that women have had and they turned out to be right!

Nell's midwifery Tutor's voice from the past rang in her ears. "Listen to what the woman tells you…if she says she is ready to push…believe her."

"How do you feel now Madge?" Nell inquired.

"I feel like I am floating away and my life blood is draining out of me," replied Madge.

The adrenaline pumped through Nell! She assessed Madge again, trying to keep calm, but her own heart rate was rising! Again she found all parameters normal. Nell read the prenatal record again, as this was not one of her own patients, incase she had missed something. She was in the Bridgeton area of Glasgow. The only thing that Nell could think of was that this baby was girl number three and they had wanted a boy this time, but Madge was cuddling the baby and they had a named her already—Ellen.

The doctor arrived and examined Madge. "All is fine Sister. You don't need me here. Why did you call me out?"

"I told the Sister that I feel I'm dying Doctor," said an eerie voice from the bed.

"Send for the flying squad, Sister," ordered the doctor. Madge had spooked him too.

The flying squad came and they agreed with Nell and the doctor that all appeared normal, but Madge kept saying, "I know that I'm dying".

The flying squad Doc hung an IV and transported Madge, with babe, to Rotten Row. She was in hospital for ten days and all was physically fine. She was discharged home. A month later Madge was diagnosed with a severe Post Partum Depression.

¤

Nell had difficulty in finding St Joseph's Place. She was doing some visits for Wendy Kelly, who was one of the Sisters in the Bridgeton area. This was a really old street that had been almost lost in the midst of new buildings.

Nell recalled Wendy saying, "You have to enter through a lane as the building is behind the main street." This whole building should have been demolished, as it was in a sorry state with small doorways and low ceilings. It was as if it had been built for the Picts (wee people), a town version of Scarra Brae. Only this had not been abandoned as it should have been, as there was always some vagrant looking for a hole in the wall to lay their head.

Wendy had also given Nell some background on Josie Hartman. Josie had been abused as a child. She left home at the age of fifteen with a man who worked in a circus. He was fifteen years her senior and he had a good position in a traveling circus. She had more stability in the traveling circus with him than she had ever had in her entire life. He was good to her but, when she was eighteen, she ran off with a young handsome clown, Neville Hartman. They ended up in Glasgow when Neville got a job in the Kelvin Hall circus for the winter season. An industrial city like Glasgow did not have a high demand for professional clowns, except during the winter season, with the pantomimes and the traveling circuses. Although the Glasgow folk would say that there was a clown up every close!

Very soon, Josie's clown was not fun to be with any more, but she stuck with him as there was no where else she felt she could go. He physically and sexually abused her. Nell had noticed the fingertip bruising on her arms and thighs…a sure sign of firm pressure from a vice-like grip. They had five children; all in care, except the baby, and Wendy did not know how long she would manage to keep the baby. Wendy had suggested to Josie that she leave her clown and she would have the help of the almoner, but Josie defended Neville vehemently. He was also a compulsive gambler. She chose this situation, with the clown who was funny at work (when he got work) and an ogre at home.

Nell finally located the correct flat and knocked on the door. It squeaked as it swung open, revealing half of a half lit hallway, with piles of old clothes on the floor. An unclean smell seemed to rise from the floor; musty decay and rancid odours hung heavily in the low-ceilinged lobby. Nell looked back into the stairwell where the wind was whistling through the broken panes of the landing window. She took a deep breath of the fresher air and called, "It's the Midwife; the Green Lady."

Silence was the loud reply. Nell knew that sometimes the tenant did not answer, incase it was the rent collector for the rent arrears, or the school board officer to see why the children were not at school, or the almoner to see the children's home conditions. The midwives were usually admitted and treated with a modicum of respect; they were viewed as non-threatening and functional at best. Nell repeated her call and added, "Sister Kelly asked me to come and see you Josie. She is out on a confinement."

There was a rustle of movement, some mumbling in low tones, then an uninviting forced voice uttered, "Come in Suster." Nell felt that the voice was really saying, "Don't bother me, go away." Nell ignored the feeling of foreboding that had hit the pit of her stomach and entered. Dante's words, "abandon all hope ye who enter here," sprung to her mind as she navigated herself through the mounds of filthy rags following where the voice had sounded. The old clothes appeared to be organized into bundles ready to go to the rag store; cash was paid for old fabric and shoes. It was so many shillings per pound weight and even more was paid for wool.

Nell pushed the door open and blinked at the light filled room. There were no curtains on the windows, only the remnants of faded beige paper roller blinds adorned the panes of rain streaked glass. There was a bed recess, with a bed adorned with a mound of bedclothes on it. An old coal range, which was smaller than the usual ranges, flickered with a few embers. A table covered in newspapers and the remnants of last night's fish and chips, bore the faint smell of vinegar, which competed for a place in the odour pool and offered the olfactory nerve some relief from the offensive stench that abounded. Yesterday morning's Daily Record was lying with the horse racing section, heavily pencil marked. A couple of sparse fireside chairs, covered in all kinds of clothing, completed the furnishings of the room.

The baby hung on Josie's arm, the tiny head and arms swayed with Josie's movement as she threw some slatey coal on the fire, causing explosive sparks for a few minutes. Josie rubbed the coal off her hand on her floral frock, unperturbed that it left huge black smears. The sink at the window had only cold water, with the old well type tap and spout that rose about a foot and turned in a lazy u-shape. This allowed for pots and kettles to be placed under it for filling.

Josie was a tall thin woman with a gaunt pale face that was devoid of expression. Her eyes appeared to be sunken by the deep dark patches that encircled them and her thin tight lips appeared ready to tremble at a moment's notice. Her demeanor shouted out, "you can't hurt me any more. I'm numb." Her mousey brown hair was disheveled and matted. There was a drawer, straddling two rickety chairs, fitted out with the folded new bright green flannelette sheet, as a makeshift bed. Sister Kelly had obviously managed to get her to do this for the baby. Josie appeared to be alone in the house. It was a single apartment with the toilet on the stair landing.

"Hello Josie, I'm Sister Dickson. Sister Kelly asked me to come and see you. I believe that you need to have your stitches removed. They must be uncomfortable when you sit down."

"Aye they wur, but he took them oot wi the breed knife last night," uttered Josie nonchalantly. "He said he didnae want tae git bloody circumcised intae the bargain."

Nell's stomach heaved! The stitches were made of a blue nylon material and Nell had noticed little bits of blue with the fish and chip wrappings! Josie lay on the bed at, Nell's request. Josie moved the mound of clothes marginally as she lay on the bed. Nell found that there was still one stitch to be removed. Nell was pleased to have the slight protection of a paper mask as the semen smell rose from the bed. It was at that moment that Nell could feel the hackles on her neck stand up…she was being watched! She cautiously ran her eye over the heap of old coats on top of the bed, which doubled as blankets, and towards the bottom of the bed, her scan met two beady brown eyes staring, mask-like, out from between two sleeves of an old coat. So this was the clown, Neville Hartman. She glared at him but did not say a word and calmly finished what she had to do. Nell tried to engage Josie in some kind of conversation but to no avail…the reason being apparent.

Nell examined the baby and left some free samples of baby milk to supplement Josie's scant milk supply. The baby was a doll-like little girl, all of five pounds three ounces. She had three wisps of blonde hair, which looped into three curls on the crown of her head. Nell commented on how pretty and cozy she looked in the little pram suit that she had on. Josie's weary eyes met Nell's and spoke a silent thanks. There was a stack of baby clothes at the bottom of the makeshift cot. Josie had made an effort.

Nell left St Joseph's Close behind, but the deprivation of Josie Hartman stayed with her. Nell's mixed emotions raged within her from revulsion to anger to melancholy to frustration. Why won't these women get up and go? Why did they stay with these clowns of men and allow themselves to be constantly abused? She walked along the road longing to go back to Josie and yell at the top of her voice, "You are worth more that ten Neville Hartmans…Josie let me take you to a safe place."

She knew that Wendy Kelly was working on this one and it would make matters much worse for Josie if Nell did anything rash. Nell slipped the green belt of her double-breasted coat through the green bakelite buckle, pulled it tight, dusted herself off, and was on her way.

Perhaps something will happen when Josie reaches a certain point, before she becomes a statistic, Nell thought. Nell remembered that when she worked at Rotten Row, there was a wee woman who came in every year to have a baby. She had six children. The staff all knew her. She was always covered in bruises; her husband had punched out one of her front teeth. The staff would say to her, "Letty leave him, you don't need to be a punch ball for anyone." She, like Josie defended the lout. "Oh he loves me and he only hits me when he's drunk!" or "He only hits me when I make him angry!"

The last time Nell saw Letty she was looking great. The gap in the front of her teeth had a tooth on a plate, and not a bruise was in sight. Nell said to her, "You look smashing Letty, did you leave him?"

"Naw hen, I took the frying pan to him when he was lying stotious and broke his jaw. He wis mortified tae tell his pals an' he hisnae hit me since. An Ah jist telt him that Am goin tae git ma tubes tied if he'll no go an git snipped. The professor here said that he wid dae that fur me, an if the Big Yin disnae like it he can lump it!"

What a change in her! Letty was not going to be abused again. Josie, on the other hand, had not known anything else but abuse and was worn down into a completely submissive state. Yet she could break this chain with a bit of help. She chose not to do that at the present time.

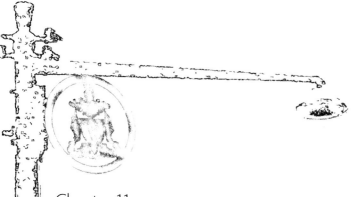

Chapter 11
Wee Sandy Stewart

"Mammy throw me doon a jeely piece, Mammy throw me doon a jeely piece…wull ye pleeeease?" Wee Sandy Stewart was yelling at the top of his voice with his innocent six year old face turned upward, so that his voice could reach the third floor of his tenement building where his Mammy was in the kitchen, and at the sink at the window, he hoped.

His wee face lit up as he saw the kitchen window open from the bottom and a white paper poke appeared at the end of an arm. Sandy watched it be tossed into the air and get bigger, as it fell towards him. He caught it with both of his arms, as he ran forward a few steps, and a big smile swept across his face, revealing a gap where his two front teeth used to be. His sandy, reddish hair was tousled and his freckles abounded. He tore into the paper poke and then "got tore" into the "piece and jam"; it had butter on it too, which made the jam moist and slippery under his tongue. He loved a jeely piece, especially when it came from above! There was something special about that. His wee pal Archie came running over to see what he was eating.

"Oh gonnae gie-us a bit Sandy I'm starvin."

"Hey Mammy," Sandy waited a few seconds to let the message reach the right mammy's ears, "gonnae gie Archie a jeely piece too?" The upturned face yelled once more, then he remembered to add, " pleeease Mammy".

Up went the window and down came another white paper poke with the treasured jeely piece in it.

The two boys sat on top of the midden wall eating their pieces and swinging their legs and trying to talk, with mouths full of Scottish plain bread, New Zealand Anchor butter and Galbraith's rhubarb and ginger jam; a pure taste of heaven! Sandy's mammy, Jessie, told him that The New Zealand butter added the goodness of sunshine to boys, in a climate that was scarce in that department. His Mammy's sister, his Aunty Sadie, lived in New Zealand, so she knew, and Sandy thought that he was an authority on that one too.

The "midden" was the brick housing for the rubbish bins for the tenement buildings, usually set behind the drying greens in the back courts and attached to the old wash houses. It was typical to have a complete block of tenement buildings facing onto four different streets, therefore, there were four rows of middens forming a quadrangle at the heart of the back courts. Each back court was separated by a brick wall or an iron railing, each possessing equal "falling off" potential.

When Nell worked in emergency, the admitting clerk, who wore her lips like Donald Duck, would be constantly wheeling in a "wee banged up boy" and saying, "another F.A.D."; "Fell Aff a Dyke" was the translation.

Nell would ask the boys, "What happened to you son?" The answer was always the same. "Ye' see, it wis like this, Ah fell aff a dyke nurse." The dyke was often the back court wall or the midden wall. These walls were high—about six feet, so it was quite a drop for the under tens.

The back court culture was unique. Although the children could not see the mothers, the mothers could see them, and with trained selective hearing, could hear them too. There would always be someone looking out. In the event of a loud piercing scream, there would be at least thirty faces at windows, looking out to see what the trouble was.

If an adult saw a child doing something wrong or dangerous, they would check them for it and if the child gave them any hassle, they would give them a swift "cuff on the lug" and say, "I'll tell your mammy if I see you doin that again." It was community parenting and it was effective.

The upward calls were continuous from the back court; "Mammy he hit me!"

"Mammy she took ma bike."

"Maw I'm hungry," and the likes.

In the summertime especially, the noise in the back courts was constant and could range from that hum of human interactions to the high pitched screeches of excitement. There was a lot of laughter too—many noises, but the music of life, never the less. At times, the calling was in reverse, going downwards.

"Sandy son come up, your dinner's ready," or "Mary hen wull you go an' get some messages for me, here's the money an' the list," and down would come a paper poke with the said contents safely tucked in it and attached to a string bag.

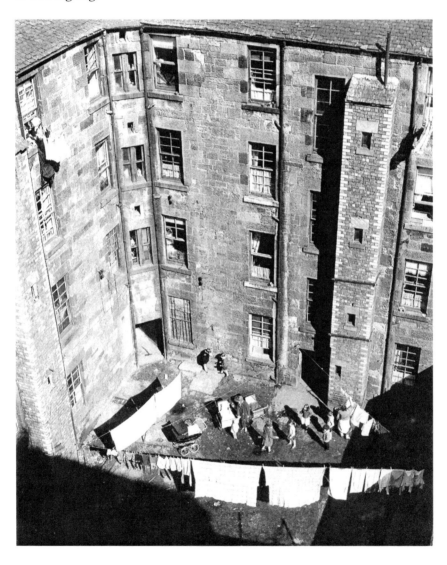

Glasgow Comedians had a field day with the back court humour. Nell often chuckled at some of the things she heard. Shouting down to the backcourt was a great direct way to communicate, not only to the intended receiver, but also to the whole back court and through all the open windows.

One standard joke was a mother shouting down to her child, "Come up for your tea, your hauf egg's ready and your faither's finished wi' the spoon."

The Salvation Army would play their Brass Band instruments in the back courts on a Sunday morning if they had permission from one of the tenants. This usually pleased about fifty percent of those within earshot.

There was little television in the 60s and the children's shows were earmarked for an hour in the afternoon and early evening. Children played in the streets or the back court. The back courts were often safer than playing in the street. Children would stage concerts and plays, and there would be the hundreds of football games on the go.

Two boys and a ball and you had a football game, and before long the players would increase. As they warmed up, their jerseys would replace the sticks or stones for goal posts. There would be games of marbles or beds (hopscotch) where an empty shoe or floor polish tin made a wonderful peever. There was many a lesson learned from playing back court games.

Sandy Stewart and Archie Murdoch had jumped down off the midden wall and decided to play a game of cops and robbers. They were scampering in and out of the old wash houses, which were great places to hide. Another two boys soon joined them in their class at school, and the game lasted for a long time, with the rules changing as they went along. Sandy tripped as he was negotiating a low broken wall and fell, letting out a blood-curdling yell. He did not fall from a great height, but his femur snapped as he twisted.

Nell was doing some relief visits in Govan and climbing the stairs to pay a post-natal visit, when she was almost knocked over by Jessie Stewart, who was flying down the stairs with a couple of towels flapping in her hands.

When she saw Nell she said, "Oh Sister, ma wean Sandy's had a bad fall." Nell turned on her heels and followed Jessie down into the back court.

Soon a group of women gathered round Jessie's wee wounded wean. If there had been someway that they could have taken the pain, these women would have. Nell examined Sandy, who now had his head on a folded towel. His mother was stroking his head with one hand and holding his wee pale hands in the other. His freckled face was ashen under the salty tearstains. His red eyes were now fixed on his Mammy. He loved his Mammy and the faces of the other mothers there were full of empathy for Jessie at that moment.

"Just you lie still Sandy and we'll get your broken leg more comfortable," Nell said. Then she turned to some of the women and said, "I'll need about eight magazines or thick newspapers and someone to phone for an ambulance. Sandy has broken his leg."

One woman said, "I'll nip intae the hairdresser's an get the magazines, that'll be the quickest."

And another offered, "I'll come wi yi Senga and phone for the ambulance from there."

Their quick wit as to the availability of what was needed was spontaneous.

In a flash, Nell had what she required to splint the leg. She slipped the glossy magazines onto one of Jessie's towels, carefully slid it under Sandy's leg, pinning the towel firmly, which created a splint, in an effort to avoid any further displacement of Sandy's broken bone. Nell had first seen this done when she was about nine years old and it was imprinted on her mind.

¤

She was out playing with her sister Agnes and some of her friends. One of the friend's wee brothers was tagging along. He was a "harum-scarum" type of boy, with long gangly arms and legs, always in mischief and pestered the girls incessantly. His mother had told his sister, his senior by one year, to mind him. He climbed on top of an information board, on which there was a map of Penilee, (which was near Nell's home). Since there was nothing to grip his sandshoes on, he lost his footing and fell off.

His leg was a funny shape, Nell remembered, and she knew that the bone was broken. They saw a district nurse in the distance and Agnes and one of her friends hared away after her shouting for help, as the others scooted off for Ian's mother. Nell stayed with Ian and he was making weird moaning sounds. The Nurse came and asked Nell to get some newspapers or books. Nell watched in awe at the way the nurse bandaged his leg. She spoke about it for months to come.

¤

Archie McCall and the other boys were looking on as Nell told Sandy what she was doing. She had safety pins in the pocket of her case and she tightened the towel round the magazine splint.

"You will have to be in hospital for a while Sandy, but you will have your mother into see you every day and your pals can see you at the weekends. Will that be OK?"

"Aye Sister," Sandy said fighting the tears.

"I know that it is sore just now, but once they get you to the hospital and put a proper splint on it won't hurt as much." Nell knew that the muscle spasm of the hamstrings in the thigh would be really painful.

"You are being very brave you know, Sandy," encouraged Nell.

Sandy replied with a toothless half-grin.

There was the sound of heavy feet coming through the close.

"Where's the wounded soldier then, you lot," joked the St. Andrew Ambulance man, as the crowd parted a path so they could clearly see wee Sandy.

"Hey! Are you no the lucky wee man wi' aw they wumin roon ye? That's never happened to me," the first ambulance man said as he winked at Sandy.

"Whit's yir name son?" said the second ambulance man.

"Sandy Stewart, Sir."

"Noo is that no jist great Hughie, did you hear the 'Sir'", he said to his partner.

"This wean'll go far. Well Sandy, we are going to take you to the Southern General Hospital in oor 'super duper' ambulance. Where's your mammy?"

"Here this is her, Sir."

"Mrs. Stewart, you go and get your things an' come wi' us in the ambulance."

"Thanks Sister for your help," Jessie said and hurried on her way.

Two women flanked her to see if they could help hold the fort while she was at the hospital.

"Thanks Sister, you have done our work for us," said the ambulanceman as he and his partner lifted wee Sandy onto a stretcher and carried him out to the waiting blue and white ambulance that had the St. Andrew's Cross on the sides. Sandy's pals were hot on their heels peering into the open ambulance. The men got Sandy settled and allowed his pals to stand inside the ambulance.

"You're dead lucky Sandy, gettin' a hurl in this," Archie said looking round the inside of the ambulance.

Sandy beamed back. His luck that day landed him in hospital for about three months on traction, but his leg would heal well. Nell had worked in that ward in the Southern General; ward eighteen, the male orthopedic ward. There were usually about six large cots at the end of the ward for the boys on traction. The men in the ward were good to them keeping them supplied with comics and goodies. The boys were aces at hanging out of the cots, almost suspended by the leg on traction, and they would scoot wee motors or comics to one another along the floor. The occupational therapist would also give them projects to work on, but they invented their own entertainment. Such was the lot of the F.A.D. and for sure, wee Sandy Stewart would miss his jeely pieces from above.

Nell straightened her coat, slipped the green belt through the green bakelite buckle, tugged to tighten it, lifted her case, and continued back up the close to her next visit.

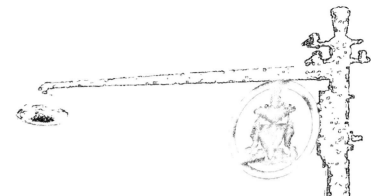

Chapter 12
Hector McCall

"Naw-al-no."
"Aye-ye-wull."
"Naw-ah-wulnae."
"By Goad ye wull lassie! Dae ye hear me? I said get doon frae there this meenit."

Reluctantly, the wee blonde headed toddler, of all of sixteen months, descended from the uppermost part of a high-backed chair. She had her face screwed up and her chin in the air. To say that she was nonplussed by the order from her Granny would be an understatement.

"That's mair like it hen," said the Granny, whose blood pressure was slowly throbbing back to normal.

"Come away an' see what I've got for you, Anne Marie," said the Granny to the huffy toddler.

"Naw-al-no," was the swift reply.

The Granny shook her head in disbelief. "That wean'll be the death o'me wi her climbing," said Granny as she walked into the bedroom where her daughter, Joan lay in bed trying to rest.

The hospital doctor had said that Joan could go home on one condition; strict bed rest. Only up to the toilet and definitely no smoking. Those were his orders. Her mother Effie, who stayed upstairs from her, said that she would help with Anne Marie and there was a maternity home help to do the washing, shopping and most of the cooking. Nell had been asked to make antenatal visits twice a week, as Joan was expecting her baby soon. The plan was for Joan to go into hospital to have her baby and aftercare, because she has a grade three cardiac condition. Joan was so upset in hospital and grieving for Anne Marie, that they let her go home.

Joan was thirty-five and did not think that she would have any family, as she had been married to Dan Spenser for eleven years before Anne Marie arrived. The doctor wanted her to have a tubal ligation so that she would not have any more babies to complicate her worsening heart condition. She had had such an easy time in labour that she definitely wanted to have another baby, against medical advice. Anne Marie was a handful, but as cute as a button and as quick as a wick. Blonde hair, big brown eyes and a petite frame, she was an absolute beauty and a climber to boot!

Joan's heart condition had suffered greatly from about the twelfth week of this pregnancy, just when she had the pregnancy confirmed. The doctors talked about an abortion, but Joan would not hear of it. It was against her Catholic religion. She was breathless on the slightest exertion. Even turning over in bed was an effort.

Nell checked the baby's heartbeat and let Joan listen through the stethoscope. She loved to listen to it.

"It's definitely a boy. I think we'll call him Daniel after his dad," Joan said smiling, "A boy'll be company for Dan."

Then she looked at Nell, with her piercing blue eyes and an all knowing look, which implied, "when I'm no longer here!"

Women who lived with compromising cardiac conditions knew the risk of childbearing. They usually had an easy time in labour, as if the body knew to take it easy, but the toll on the heart and circulation was so great that many of them did not live to see the baby reach two months of age. After delivery, they were not given the usual medication to control the bleeding. If they have a large blood loss, it reduced the load on the heart and the medication could increase their blood pressure.

"Well, be it he or she, the heartbeat is regular anyway," said Nell smiling with something positive to say. "Sounds like a big pocket watch ticking ten to the dozen."

"Ma' doctor comes tae see me every day. He made arrangements wi' the hert doctor and the obstetrician frae ra' hoaspital. Then they speak on ra phone about ma pills an' that."

"You are in the best of hands. You have three good men looking after you," reassured Nell.

"Aye Ah hiv that, an Ah jist hope that I pull through fur them."

"Mammy look whit Granny gied me," Anne Marie came chargin' in with a pop up book.

"Sit up here, hen an A'll read it tae yi," said Joan.

"OK Mammy!" and Anne Marie climbed on the bed gently as though she sensed the frailty of her mother's condition.

Nell smiled and waved goodbye. "See you on Tuesday, Joan."

"Aye then Sister, ma' Ma will see yi tae the door."

"Cheerio Anne Marie," but Anne Marie was showing her Mammy how the pop-up book worked.

"Oh see 'at Mammy yi' jist dae it like this."

Nell wiped a tear away from her cheek as she went down the stairs. The picture of mother and daughter lingered with her and kept popping into her consciousness throughout the day. The drive for women to have a baby when the odds are so against them was a phenomenal thing; that biological clock had a powerful tick at times. Nell prayed that Joan would pull through, but she knew that the reason she was allowed home from hospital was to spend as much quality time with Anne Marie as possible, as there was not much more they could do for her. So often these women died from heart complications about five weeks after delivery. Would there be a miracle for Joan?

Nell was doing some post partum visits for another midwife who was on holiday. These visits were in the Oatlands area of Glasgow's south side. She knocked on Mrs. Stevenson's door and to her great surprise, Hector McCall opened it. His face said it all! He did not want Maisie to know about this. Nell thought that he was playing around, as she had smelled the faint scent of "Evening in Paris" perfume off him the night the twins were born.

"Hello. I'm filling in for Sister Laidlaw," said Nell, not mentioning that she knew Hector.

"Come in Sister, you will find your patient in the kitchen. I'm off then, Flo."

"Oh Hecky, before you go can you take them pills back to the chemist, they're the wrang wans."

Hector was forced to go into the kitchen where Flora Stevenson gave him the pills and a peck on the cheek. "Thanks Hecky, see yi later then, remember yir key."

All he said in reply was "aye" and he was off, closing the door firmly behind him and wishing the floor could have swallowed him up.

Flora Stevenson was a pleasant, attractive woman and at least fifteen years older than Hector. She was one of his sister's friends and so he had often been in her house at parties and gatherings. The Stevenson parties were a regular occurrence. She was married to a Merchant Seaman, Chuck, who sailed with the British India Steam Navigation Company (B.I.). Nell remembered the black and white funnels of the B.I. Ships from her primary School days. Chuck would be away from home up to ten months at a time on the Calcutta/Bombay run.

Flora was tall and lean with shiny black hair and light brown eyes. She had one son, Gordon, who was twelve years old and she had been desperately trying to get pregnant each time Chuck was home, but she had several miscarriages. She wasn't getting any younger and felt that her biological clock was ticking faster.

Hector had been at one of Flora's parties with his sister, not long after Chuck had sailed. He got too drunk to walk home and had crashed on the sofa to sleep it off a bit. As he came to, he found Flora making a move on him. Somehow, he was lying on his side, in her bed, naked. She was lying behind him with an arm drenched over his hip. He froze with the realization of his strange surroundings. He would creep out and home to Maisie. What had he done in his drunken state? He usually was useless till he sobered up. That's what Maisie always said.

Oh God! Oh God! Please help me sneak away out of this nightmare! He pinched his leg to make sure he was awake.

Hector moved his top leg towards the edge of the bed and felt Flora's arm fall on the bed.

She must be asleep, he surmised. So far so good.

Then he rolled his shoulders that way too. Good, she must still be asleep.

Inch by inch, he eased himself towards the edge of the bed.

Great, he was sitting up now and his feet were firmly on the floor. His mouth was dry and his heart was pounding. He did not dare to look behind him. Now where were his clothes? Oh where were his clothes? Maisie, I love you! I wish I was with you at this moment. I'm so stupid at times!

No clothes in sight, perhaps they were in the other room? All was still in the twilight, nothing was moving except his heart, which was now pounding in his throat and battering his eardrums. He panted noiselessly through his open, arid mouth. He reached for the door handle, turned and tugged it, turned and tugged again, twisted it the other way and tugged it. It did not budge. It was bloody well locked! What's this all about? He turned round and looked toward the bed, shielding his nakedness with his large freckly hands.

There she lay, in a scanty black silk negligee, her shoulders and face pale against its blackness, her slim arms long and empty. Her silky black hair framed her face like a picture. Her eyes closed, lips ruby red and as he looked at the lips, they broke into a smile and her eyes opened wide.

"Where do you think you are going, lover boy?"

"I'm going home to Maisie, and I'm not your lover boy!" exclaimed Hector.

"That's not the way you acted last night, Hecky," replied Flora.

"I don't believe you, because Maisie says that I'm useless when I'm drunk."

"Perhaps to Maisie, but definitely not to me, Hecky."

"I want my clothes, where are they Flo?"

"Oh poor boy needs his clothes," she pouted as she spoke the words. "Well I'll give them to you, on one condition."

"Aye and what may that be?" Hector asked, the highland brogue being more noticeable with his rising agitation.

"Come here and I'll tell you," she said as she patted the cream coloured silken sheets.

Hector sat on the bed like a sulking child and she knelt up behind him, rubbing his shoulders in a rhythmic sway. She then swung herself astride him and kissed the top of his head holding his head closely to her breasts. He put his hands on the bed behind him to steady himself. Then she sat on his naked lap and he felt her warmth on him. Gently she pushed him on to his back.

She massaged him and whispered in his ear, "I need a baby before Chuck comes back and I need to get pregnant now, so he thinks it is his. Come on Hecky, you have plenty to spare. This will be our secret, once only. I promise. I couldn't miss a chance like this with Gordon staying with his Granny this weekend. I know you will enjoy it big time; I'll make sure you do."

She began to get a bit rougher with him in her eagerness. He rose to the occasion and swung her on to her back and they had intercourse with Flora calling out to him in encouragement, "At a boy! Keep it up! Go for gold! You're the winner!" He had never experienced that before. A bit disconcerting to say the least, but he did deliver the goods.

He didn't dislike the event, although he felt like a hired stud. It had been different and exciting in a way, he must admit. She made him a big nosh-up of bacon, eggs and sausages and fried potato scones, lashings of tea and a mountain of toast. Hector feasted. He went home to Maisie satisfied and his tail between his legs!

He dropped in on Flora the next day in the early afternoon before Gordon was home from school. Flora went straight to the bedroom and began stripping off.

She shouted, "What's keeping you? We only have an hour before Gordon is home from school."

"Oh I only came in to see if you are pregnant, are you?"

"Come on Hecky, you know it is not as simple as that. You can give me double the chance though."

She was handing him this on a plate. No strings attached. Many a man would jump at the chance. He would turn her on today, so that she could see what he was made of. He did not need the cheering squad today.

"Right Flora, are you ready for this?"

He knelt on the bed beside her and disrobed her, softly caressing her neck and hair as he did so. He sat behind her on the bed, with a leg out on each side of her and fondled her breasts, taking the nipples between two fingers and stroking them.

She lay back against him, like putty in his hands, responding with hip movements when he flicked her nipples. With one hand on her breast, the other easily reached down between her legs and fondled the top of each leg. Her body arched against him, and then he moved his hand to her groin, left then right, now on the pubic bone where he rubbed his fingers in a circular motion. His other hand tweaked each erect nipple and she rocked her pelvis to encourage his fingers towards the already pulsating clitoris. It was a macho thing; he was in control this time and she whimpered as he masterfully made love. No cheering was necessary. They both lay quietly in the afternoon light; there was no need for words.

She thought, "No wonder Maisie has so many weans," and he thought, "I'll need tae tell big Duncan that they French films work."

Hector was a most welcomed visitor with fancy sex and big nosh-ups, until the pregnancy was confirmed. Then Flora became out of bounds. She had what she wanted. She did not want to lose this pregnancy as she had done before. It was precious to her. Hector did a few odd jobs around the house for her and looked in on her now and again.

When the baby was born, his curiosity could not be quelled. He had to see Flora's baby. There she was, a six pound pink bundle of joy with red curly hair and looked just like the McCall twins. But then, so did hundreds of babies in Scotland and Hector had not been near their mothers!

Nell performed the postnatal visit. She lifted Sarah out of her cot.

"What a cherub you are with those red curls," Nell commented.

"Yes. My husband Chuck's mother had red hair, so we called her after her. Her hair is white now, of course. They do say that red hair misses a generation. Is that not right, Sister?"

"Yes it can, then there are some that pass it on directly too."

End of the red hair story, thought Nell, as long as the McCall twins and Sarah Stevenson don't end up in the same class at school. Nell was sure that thought had crossed Flora's mind too.

"You, Sarah my girl," said Nell, examining the baby, "have lovely smooth skin for a three week post mature baby." Flora had given the expected date a month before it actually was.

"Yes!" said Flora, "She has peaches and cream complexion just like my sister's girls and her Daddy can't wait to see her. He has bought up the toy store in Hong Kong for her."

Hector would have to stop dropping in on Flora now, as her husband was due home soon. Flora had burned the result of Chuck's poor sperm count result. She phoned the clinic to say that they were moving and that they were not going to pursue it any more, so to close the file. Chuck did not need to know that now. It does something to a man's morale, Flora thought, to know that his sperm count is below normal. She did love Chuck and hoped that he would be home for a long leave this time.

Nell hoped that things worked out for the Stevenson family.

The biological clock was a strong motivator! Nell put on her double-breasted coat and slipped the belt through the green bakelite buckle, picked up her case and was, once again, on her way.

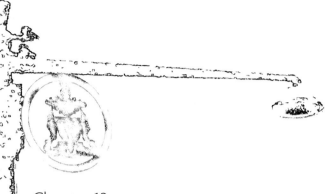

Chapter 13
Ruby Singleton

The Singletons were a large family with twelve children now; mother Meg and father Matt, three dogs, two cats and a budgie. They lived in Gorbals. They had, in fact, two flats, side by side on one landing, and had knocked a door way through to inter connect, which gave them six rooms in total and two toilets. This was unheard of in flats in Glasgow at that time.

Nell had just delivered the last baby, who made the seventh girl. A heavenly number, Nell jested. The placenta was delivered and Nell, as usual, laid it in the ashet pie dish and put it to the side.

Suddenly Rex, the dog, swooped by and stole the placenta, knocking the enameled ashet to the floor. The dish landed with spluttering bangs as the dog ran off leaving a trail of blood behind him! Consternation ruled! Three of the Singleton children ran after him, yelling at the top of their voices, but the placenta was gone; eaten by Rex! The other dogs were close in pursuit and were licking up the blood that had been spilled in the retreat. Nell had heard of this happening, but this was the first time that she had experienced it. Well that was one placenta that she could not examine for completeness. She would have to keep that in mind as, if any placenta was left in the uterus and not expelled, it could lead to infection and hemorrhage.

Meg Singleton was thirty-nine and her eldest child was sixteen. She did not have many problems in childbearing. She said it was too easy and she handled her children well. The family was her pride and joy. Meg had a good sense of humour and she certainly needed it. This was the second baby that Nell had delivered for Meg. She delivered Bobby almost two years ago. Meg said then that she would probably have another to round off the numbers and she did; but it made them more uneven! Seven girls and five boys was the final total. Meg confided to Nell that this was definitely the last one and she was going to call her Margaret Rose after herself and Princess Margaret.

"An' Ah'll no let them shorten it to Meg like ma Ma did to me Sister."

Margaret Rose junior weighed nine pounds. She had rosy cheeks and was as bald as a coot, although if you looked closely, there was fine white hair all over her scalp. Meg now had five children under six years old. The older children were good at looking after the younger ones. If they didn't do that then their mother didn't get the cooking, washing and shopping organized.

Matt Singleton was a hard-working man, who was employed in a Clyde-side galvanizing plant. The Company was famous for their galvanized lampposts. He was a foreman there and had good steady money coming in, which was just as well with all the mouths to be fed and feet to be shod. Meg had been a French polisher in the shipyards before she fell pregnant and had never worked since having Paul, the eldest boy. They both had had the chance to stay at school till they were eighteen and wanted their children to do the same. It was hard leaving school at fifteen and scrambling to get an apprenticeship or being the tea boy or girl for a year, waiting on an opportunity to move onto the next slippery rung of the labour ladder.

The Singleton parents realized that a good education would go a long way to aid their children's future careers, so they encouraged reading and drawing and made sure that the homework was done. The seventh child in the family was Ruby. Ruby was a small child for her age with long blonde pigtails and hazel coloured eyes. She had a quiet manner and gave her mum a hand with the younger siblings who were all robust and big for their ages, yet Ruby carried them about. If Ruby was not helping her mum with the wee ones, she could be found sitting quietly in a corner with her nose in a library book; reading was her passion. She had never been a problem to her parents. In actual fact, none of the Singletons gave their parents any extra worry. The parents were respected. Meg Singleton found out one day that Ruby was a "gifted" child; she recounted the happenings that day to Nell.

A new teacher had come to the school and spotted Ruby's giftedness right away. The young teacher was so excited about this that she asked Ruby to bring her mother back with her after lunch. This was when Meg was about eleven weeks pregnant and she was having terrible morning sickness that lasted almost all day.

In came Ruby from school and said, "Mammy you've got tae come back to the school wi' me. The teacher said you huv tae."

Meg was worried that Ruby had done something wrong. Although she felt like death warmed up, and still felt nauseated with a frontal headache and longed for a lie down, she gathered up the four children under five, bundled then into the large deep pram and bounced it down the stairs. With each bounce the toddlers shrieked with delight as the airborne wheels landed on the next step. The pram was well sprung, so it gave two or three bounces each time. The shrieks of delight and the chorus high-pitched voices yelling "dae nat again Mammy," seemed to ricochet off the inside walls of Meg's skull. She was concentrating on keeping hold of the pram and its precious cargo.

Thank God we only live on the first floor, Meg thought, as she reached the ground floor.

Mrs. Seaton opened her door on the ground level to see what the noise was all about. The older lady smiled at the happy faces, but a concerned looks swept over her when she looked directly at Meg.

"Meg, are you OK hen? You look awffy peely wally."

"I'll be OK, Ah just huv tae go up to the school a minnit wi' Ruby," Meg replied.

"When yi get back Ah'll come up an' let yi get a wee lie doon, OK?" Mrs. Seaton said reassuringly.

"That's awffy good o' you Mrs. Seaton. Ah canny deny that that's what Ah'm need," said Meg.

"Here wait a minnit an Ah'll gei the weans a wee treat," Mrs. Seaton said.

Momentarily, Mrs. Seaton was back with a tin of Cadbury's chocolate fingers. She gave them each two fingers, except for ten-month old Bobby, who was miraculously asleep amid the chaos.

"That'll keep them quiet for a wee while. I'll watch out for yi getting back hen," said Mrs. Seaton.

"Thanks Mrs. Seaton," replied Meg.

"Ocht jist ca me Bessie."

"Right yi are then, Bes. Bessie," Meg responded shyly.

Meg was uncomfortable calling her elders by their first name; something that had been hammered into her as a child.

Mrs. Seaton had been in that house all her married life. She was now in her early eighties and had raised four children, two boys and two girls. She was an active octogenarian and never let things get her down. She was fond of Meg and loved the biz and buzz of the Singleton children. Some older people hated noise, but she never complained.

Perhaps the Singletons made up for her lack of grandchildren. Bessie Seaton's two boys immigrated to South Africa after the war. They both married but neither of them had any family. They always sent their mother a parcel on her birthday and at Christmas. Bessie's oldest daughter immigrated to America and she was married with one daughter. She came to visit her mother periodically, but always stayed in a hotel in Glasgow. Bessie's younger daughter had multiple sclerosis and died tragically at the age of twenty-two. Mr. Seaton had been a carpet buyer and died of lung cancer when he was seventy.

Bessie's home was comfortable with nice pieces of antique furniture and old, but good, Persian rugs. She had a large grandfather clock in the hallway. The Singleton children loved to watch the pendulum swing as it made a loud tick. The clock had a booming chime every fifteen minutes and the children got quite excited if they heard the clock gearing up for a chime.

The children echoed a chorus of "ta" for the biscuits from Mrs. Seaton and straightway "got tore" into the chocolate fingers. The twin two-year-olds, Alec and Alice, seemed to spread the chocolate right round their entire faces. The three and a half year old Mary was patiently licking the chocolate off each and every finger in turn; a methodically painstaking exercise. When the pram would bounce over a stone her tongue would lick air and the chocolate finger would smear her chin and she would giggle. It began to spit with rain as the troupe proceeded up towards the school. As they approached the bell was ringing.

"Who's dongin' the bell Mammy?"

"Let me see, Ah canny see ra' bell Mammy."

"Can Ah ring the bell Mammy?"

The questions were incessant.

"Wheesht a wee minnit," said Meg as she was straining to listen to Ruby directing her where to go.

"OK hen, you go to your line an Ah'll come in tae see yir teacher in a wee minnit. Oh! Ruby whit's her name again hen?" asked Meg.

"Miss Anderson, Mammy, and its room nine," said Ruby clearly and smiling at her Mammy at the same time. She was pleased and excited that her mammy was coming to see her nice teacher.

"Right 'o Ruby hen, see you soon then," said Meg.

Meg watched Ruby join her class line, which marched in twos into the class.

As Meg stood under the playground shelter with the big pram, shielding the wee ones from the light rain, watching Ruby's line disappear, she could not help thinking how small Ruby was in comparison to some of the other girls there. Still, she seemed to like this class and school and there had never been any problem with her schoolwork. Till now.

Well I better go and see what the problem is, thought Meg.

She pulled her coat to straighten it but didn't notice that it was buttoned up crookedly. Her silky headscarf was a bit wet, clinging to her head like a clam, but it would have to do. She still felt a bit nauseated and headachy.

She wiped the rain off her "National Health" glasses and suddenly wished that they did not have an obvious cracked lens with the discoloured elastoplast holding the right leg secure. She would get a new pair of glasses in the summer, when she would have more time to go and see the optician.

She pushed the pram determinedly over to the door of the school and helped the three wee ones to disembark. They were all dressed in knitted hats, wee velvet collared tweed coats (which buttoned to the waist), knee length socks and sturdy black polished lacing shoes. The hand-me-down coats had been well washed in their day, but still regained their shape, although the velvet on the collars was pretty flat. The two elder brothers had polished all the shoes; that was their evening chore. When they finished, their dad inspected the "Dubbin" polish. The Dubbin helped to make the seams on the leather shoes waterproof. Sturdy shoes and good food were priorities in the Singleton household.

Meg looked at her three children, as they stood all agog, swallowing up all they saw. They were in awe of "the big school" and quiet with it. Long may that remain, Meg thought.

The three children were covered in Mrs. Seaton's chocolate fingers. The smirring of rain had augmented the spread of the chocolate to reach more of their hands, faces, coats and legs. She tried in vain to clean them up with a bit of spit and the corner of her cotton pinny. She put the brake on the pram and lifted baby Bobby out. He was a big armful—ten months and twenty-two pounds! He was warm and cozy and red-faced and "hummin'" with a newly laid full nappy load, and what a pong! Well there is no turning back now, thought Meg.

"Right, right kids: Mary, Alex, Alice, stay wi me noo and don't touch anything. Keep nice and quiet will yi?"

"Aye Mammy Ah wull," chorused the reply.

"Remember yi're in the big School." That seemed to have a quieting effect on the little characters.

Room nine appeared! Meg squinted through the cracked lens, as the uncracked wet lens was steaming up with the warmth of the school's central heating. She knocked on the door amid the glaur of chocolate, with its lingering sweet smell mixing with the unmistakable baby fecal odour!

"Mrs. Singleton, is it?"

Meg nodded in reply.

"Thank you so much for coming. I'm Letty Anderson," and a hand was offered to shake.

As Meg shook her hand, baby Bobby went up and down with the hand shake, which had the effect of wafting the pungent odour further. Ensuring that, not one olfactory receptor in a ten feet radius was left unscathed by the pungent putrid odour!

Meg smiled and had a look at this fresh sweet teacher all of twenty-two if she was a day. She was a brunette, nice build, eyes that seemed to sparkle, and a wide-open smile showing off perfect white teeth. She was dressed in a beige ribbed jumper that hugged a thirty-four B bust, a brown belted mini-ish skirt and high brown leather boots. She looked well coordinated and Meg instinctively liked her. What had her lassie done!

"What's Ruby done, Miss Anderson?" asked Meg.

"Oh Ruby isn't in trouble, Mrs. Singleton. I feel that Ruby is a gifted child; like a child genius and I would like to get your permission to have her tested by an Educational Psychologist. I have spoken to the headmaster and he would like to see you. If we don't keep her interested she will get very bored and not achieve her potential," explained Miss Anderson.

Meg stood there with her mouth wide open, her glasses had now totally steamed up, her head scarf had been pulled to one side by the monster baby in her arms, revealing a couple of 'dainty' metal hair curlers in the mass of flattened straw coloured hair. The three wee ones were grasping the hem of her coat where a unique chocolate 'fingered' pattern was emerging. Meg tried to absorb that her Ruby was a genius. She closed her mouth. She felt so glaekit and said, "Of course! Whatever is best for Ruby, Miss Anderson."

Meg found herself sitting in front of Mr. Dick, the headmaster. An assistant had taken the three wee ones into an adjoining room and given them juice and biscuits and a selection of toys, which were a big draw. Meg still had her arms full of one smelly big baby who had now decided to be shy and bury his head in Meg's neck, which quickly became covered in slobber.

Mr. Dick told Meg that they would have Ruby tested by an Educational Psychologist and depending on that report they would like to offer her special classes and perhaps music lessons too, on whatever musical instrument she would like.

Meg thanked him very much and once again that afternoon gathered her brood about her and headed home. Somehow the drink of juice and the news at the school had cleared her headache. Mrs. Seaton did come up and let Meg have a "wee doss"; it was the sweetest sleep filled with floating music and Ruby in fine clothes. Imagine her wee Ruby a genius; a real gem she was.

The results of the tests proved that Ruby was gifted in all disciplines. She received lots of extra schoolwork. Nell could hear Ruby playing the piano. Up and down the scales she went in perfect timing. Her Dad was so proud of her that he had managed to buy a piano from an old lady that Mrs. Seaton knew. Ruby shared what she learned and had already taught one of her older brothers the basics of the piano. He wanted to play the guitar. She had a green sticker on the key of middle C, and the wee ones would show off that they could find middle C and then play, *"I am C, middle C, skip a note and go to E"*. When Nell first called to see Meg, each child had to show her how they could play it, striking the keys hard with each word they sang.

Meg and Matt were pleased to see that the extra attention had not spoiled Ruby and that she always had time for her family. Ruby would play all the nursery rhymes for the children, the *Holy City* for her Daddy and *Bless this House* for her Mammy. Mrs. Seaton would scour the second hand shops for sheet music or walk down to Allans in Calton Place on Clyde Side and find her a nice piece of music to play. Mrs. Seaton's favourite piece was called *Passing By* and Ruby played it for her. It was all about a man who loved a lady but he only ever saw her passing by. Ruby wondered why he never stopped her and spoke to her.

> *'There is a Lady sweet and kind*
> *Was never face so pleased my mind*
> *I did but see her passing by*
> *Yet will I love her till I die'*

There was always music in the Singleton's house because of one little girl and loving parents who did not want to stand in her way. Nell loved to visit the Singleton's place as the children were given pride of place and each was treated as an individual.

Meg would say, "Do you know what our Alex did the day," and before long another child would brag about what their sibling could do and not always about what they could do. There seemed to be a family pride in each other that Meg and Matt had continually fostered. It often made Nell misty and regained her faith in human nature. She always felt the better having visited the Singleton household.

Meg had confided in Nell one day to say that she was going to have her tubes tied after her sixth baby. She felt that she could not cope with any more children, but her mother became ill and she had to look after her, and consequently she did not get the sterilization operation. A month after her mother died, she found out that she was pregnant with Ruby.

"They both had a ruby for their birth stone, so we called her Ruby an' Ah hope Ah'll be able to buy her a ruby ring for her twenty first birthday." Meg shared.

"I'm sure you will Meg," assured Nell. "That will be very special for her."

"Aye she's a good one, ma Ruby."

Thanks to Bessie Seaton, who promoted Ruby, she was often invited to play the piano at Church socials both in the Protestant and Catholic churches. The neighbour-hood was proud of Ruby.

¤

Ruby Singleton was the dux of her school. She won scholarship after scholarship and went to Glasgow University. She played the piano and the cello and was part of a string quartet at Glasgow University, but she did not make music her career. It was a wonderful day for the whole family when Ruby graduated with a doctoral degree in Medicine and was one of Glasgow's first female Research Biochemists. All the family went to her graduation and, of course, Bessie Seaton did too. They all got new outfits and her mother and Bessie wore new, feathered hats. Then they all walked from the University down to Charing Cross to have a special fish diner in the Berkley Restaurant near the Mitchell Library. This had been the restaurant that Matt had first taken Meg to on their first date, many moons before.

Ruby did receive a ruby ring for her twenty-first birthday from her mother and father and she treasured it greatly. She was able to help her siblings out financially with their further education and the big hummin' baby Bobby became a family doctor, much to the family's surprise and delight.

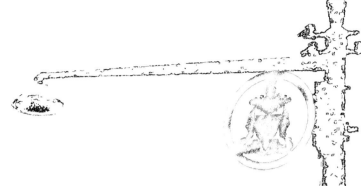

Chapter 14
Tilda: A Slip of the Tongue

Nell was sitting with her right hand on Tilda Blackie's abdomen and her left hand holding a large gent's pocket watch, her eyes following the seconds hand as it silently jerked its way round the analog face; she was intent on timing Tilda's contractions. Her hand sensed the strength, duration, and frequency of each contraction. It took time to do this thoroughly. After about fifteen minutes, she listened in to the foetal heart with the Pinnard stethoscope, which was commonly called the "trumpet" because of its shape. She listened through three contractions, timing the foetal heart with Big Bessie (what she called her gent's watch).

This was a marathon labour. If Tilda had been in hospital, they would call it "inordinate uterine action". In other words, the uterus hasn't got its act together! This may happen when the baby's head is tilted and the egg shape of the head is not central. That was one of the few drawbacks of a home confinement; when there was a drawn out labour, the midwife, by law, was tied up for the duration.

In hospital, a midwife could be spelled from these tedious situations by relief staff. Nell had managed to go out for a fish supper, to a chippie at the corner last evening, when she had the student midwife with her. The student midwife went on to another confinement about 9 p.m. The families were always offering food and drink, but Nell liked to provide her own as much as possible and always carried emergency supplies of little packets of nuts and raisins. Scottish hospitality was abundant and they would do without to give to the midwife. Many families were barely surviving on the bread line and Nell was acutely aware of this. There was a china cup with red roses on it that appeared, "for the Sister's tea," at every confinement in one particular old tenement building in Gorbals.

Tilda lived in the Pollokshaws area and her own midwife was on holiday. Tilda was happy it was Nell that had answered her call, as she had met Nell before at the Health Clinic. It was always a bonus for the mother to have met the midwife before the confinement. Nell had arrived yesterday at 3 p.m. and it was now 2 a.m.

Charlie was fussing over Tilda, fetching cold drinks, rinsing out cold cloths for her brow, getting a fresh nighty for her and helping her change into it. He also stoked up the coal fire. Charlie was being a busy bee.

Eva, the neighbour, was helping hold the fort. She had put Tilda's two daughters to bed and done the washing up. Then she made a big pot of soup, cooked up minced beef with onions and carrots and peeled potatoes ready for the mince and tatties for tomorrow's dinner. Then Eva made some girdle soda scones and offered scones and tea to everybody.

"These are my favourite scones," said Charlie. "Ma ma used to make a big batch on a Saturday morning and me and ma brothers would scoff them when we came hame frae the fitba."

The smells of all the cooking permeated the house. They were joking with Tilda that the smell of the scones would bring the baby. Nell's eye was on the second hand of the watch and she knew for sure that it would take more than the smell of the scones to bring out this wee current bun!

One positive thing was that the contractions were still happening. Tilda had one strong one, then two weak ones, similar to a posterior position labour, Nell thought. But she was sure that this baby was in a good position, except for the head, which was probably deflexed or tilted to the side. Nell had given Tilda some pethidine and she had relaxed well between the strong contractions and even snoozed through some of the weak ones. Now it was time, Nell felt, to change her position, get her up to walk about and crouch on all fours with the contractions. She could also spend some time in a warm bath (this house did have a bath).

Nell remembered the longest labour she had ever experienced. The doctor had come out and spent two hours on his knees with the woman with a similar labour pattern to Tilda's. He explained that the baby's head was trying to descend, but kept moving from side to side as if it was watching a Wimbledon tennis match, and no progress was being made. He encouraged the woman to squat and go on all fours and eventually the baby's head began the descent. Nell gave her counter back pressure and massage to ease the pain. She remembered, too, that the baby had two big bumps on its head and looked as if he had a heart shaped head. This had been caused by the baby's head rotating from side to side against the inside of the pelvis, creating friction on the skull bones. The medical term for this is bilateral cephalhaematomas, which would disappear in about six weeks. In essence it was bruising under the coverings of the skull bones.

Tilda's waters hadn't broken yet, so Nell thought that the bath would be a good start. She checked with Charlie to see if there was plenty of hot water before suggesting the bath, or to use a new term for a bath during labour, "aqua therapy". There was a movement from the "Granola Bunch" who were the back to nature folk, flower people, hippies or whatever they wanted to be called, to promote the sexuality of childbearing. It certainly was a "labour of love" for the parents and the midwife. Nell doubted if any mother would, after a 24-hour labour, call it a sexual experience, although it was a unique and wonderful experience for sure when they look into the eyes of their newborn baby. The Granola Bunch thought that they had invented "natural childbirth" and thought that women should not have medical intervention in labour. One thing that they did not realize was the fact that Homo sapiens have the poorest record in the Animal Kingdom at reproduction. Nell remembered that from one of her first lectures in her midwifery training.

"Come on Tilda and have some aqua therapy," Nell said.

"Some whit? Dae Ah huv tae drink it?" said Tilda turning up her nose.

"No. It's the new natural childbirth name for a bath in labour."

"Is that so…Aye an that loat think they've invented weans and watter!"

They all roared with laughter at the new term as Nell helped Tilda wauchle through to the bathroom. Laughter was good. It released endorphins from the brain, relieved tension and defused taught situations. Glasgow wit is an integral part of every Glaswegian. Where you get two or more Glaswegians chatting on almost any subject, it won't take very long before there is laughter. It may be the turn of phrase or the way that a story is related or witty off the cuff remarks, the humour will out, albeit self effacing. Charlie was there in front of them, filling the bath and ensuring that it wasn't too hot and supplying the towels and a couple of face cloths.

My, Nell thought, what a considerate husband!

"Does that make me the aqua therapist hen?" he asked Tilda, and they all laughed again.

Out of the bath, then sitting astride a chair, then walking up and down supported by the valiant Charlie, then crouching on all fours before Tilda suddenly became quite panicky and called out in pain. Transition at last, Nell thought! She checked Tilda with an internal exam and was pleased to report to one and all that it was almost time for this baby to descend into the world.

The contractions came one after the other, with very little rest between them. Just as suddenly as the panic had started, the contractions calmed down to one every three minutes. Nell surmised that this was now second stage, where Tilda's cervix had fully dilated and an unobstructed descent was now possible. It was clear to Nell now. Midwives knew the stage of labour without even checking the cervix. They were "at one with the woman", empathizing her feelings, picking up on her vibes and using her eyes, hands and expertise.

The pushing began and Tilda decided that she wanted to stand and deliver. She was hot and decided to strip naked. Charlie got behind her and supported her under her oxters (the armpits) with a small towel over each arm, while Nell and Eva helped at the sides. Nell had no sooner put a large towel on the floor when Tilda's waters broke with the escape of a large slurp of straw coloured fluid. Nell immediately checked the foetal heart; she was on her knees with the trumpet to Tilda's abdomen and big Bessie on a chain hanging from her pocket over her plastic apron.

The foetal heart rate was slow after the contraction, but picked up a bit to 108 beats per minute before the next contraction hit. Nell stayed on the floor, as the show was thick and heavy and Nell knew that the head was descending quickly. She asked Charlie how he was doing holding Tilda and he said "OK Sister," but he looked a bit red in the face.

"Let's move back a bit so the Charlie can be supported by the wall," Nell said.

The group shuffled backwards about a foot.

Charlie nodded thanks to Nell.

Eva was helping to take Tilda's weight too. Soon the baby's head began to appear and Nell tried to increase the flexion of the baby's head to allow the egg shaped crown to be born slowly.

"Another slow push with the next contraction, Tilda and the head will be born," Nell encouraged.

"OK Sister here it comes, Oh my Goad ahhhhhh," Tilda groaned as she reddened in the face and pushed.

"Pant now," said Nell as she eased the baby's head out through the vaginal opening and slipped her finger in to feel if there was any cord round the baby's neck. Yes! There it was, at least twice round the neck. Nell looked at the wee blue face that was motionless and picked up her two pairs of artery forceps. Quickly she clamped the cord under the baby's chin, then swiftly took her scissors and cut the cord between the two clamped forceps. A spurt of blood hit her apron and she unwound the cord from the baby's neck; three times she unwound. Tilda's eyes glared at the cord as Nell unwound it from the baby's neck.

"Now Tilda give me one last push." Nell positioned her hands to deliver the shoulders.

"Grrrrrrahhhhh, Oh Mammy Daddy! Oh Mammy Daddy! Ahhi ahhi ahhi…" and the sounds diminished from Tilda as the baby's body was born.

"It's a boy!" said Nell clearly as Tilda slumped into Charlie's arms.

The baby needed stimulation and Tilda needed attention.

Nell called instructions to Charlie and Eva to roll Tilda onto the bed on her side and hold her chin forward.

"She has just fainted," said Nell hoping that that was all it was.

"Don't worry sister I'll take care of her," Charlie said with confidence. "Ave goat ma First Aid certificate."

Nell turned her attention fully to the baby. The heart rate was twenty-five for five seconds. That was OK. No respirations, face blue, baby had some tone…Nell decided to do mouth to nose and mouth breathing. She suctioned the baby's nose and mouth with the DeLee suction catheter, then gave three small puffs into the baby's nose and mouth. Babies are obligatory nose breathers and can't easily breathe through their mouths, so it is best and easier to cover both.

Nell checked the baby's apex heartbeat again…still 100 beats per minute.

He is just taking his time, Nell thought…give more stimulation, come on baby…expand your lungs…she rubbed with a dry hot towel…Finally, the baby grimaced and his top lip curled as he breathed in, in a gasp, and breathed out in his first faint cry.

Thank you, God and two minutes exactly, Nell prayed under her breath, as she checked her watch. She noticed the large cephalhaematoma on the right side of the baby's head as she renewed the warm wrap round the baby and gave him to Eva to hold.

Now for Tilda, who had come round. Charlie had her supported on two pillows now and covered her with a sheet and wool blanket. She looked pale and distant.

"Is the wean OK Sister?" Tilda asked quietly.

"Yes he is fine and he recovered well from having the cord three times round his neck," reassured Nell. "Listen to the noise of him now."

Master Derek Blackie was crying lustily in Eva's arms.

"Whit aboot the bump oan his heed?" Tilda said.

"That will disappear in about six weeks. Remember I said he might have a bump on his head?" said Nell, "The doctor will give him a good exam later today. Keep in mind that the bump is on the outside of the bone so it is far away from the brain."

"OK then Sister," said a relieved Tilda.

While Nell and Tilda had been talking Nell was checking Tilda's blood pressure and pulse and her abdomen.

"Now let's see if the afterbirth is ready to come away," said Nell.

The confinement completed, Nell began to get the things ready to bath the baby and Eva was making breakfast. The smell of bacon sizzling in the pan and the happy chatter brought the girls through to see their new brother. Climbing on the bed they were draped over Tilda. Charlie, as protective as ever, was cautioning them not to lean on Tilda too hard.

"Look Mammy he's holding ma finger tight."

"Aw look at his wee tongue."

Nell loved to hear the comments from the siblings. Ann and Mary were seven and five years old respectively. They sat down to watch Nell bath Derek, and Charlie, beaming proudly, looked on too.

There seemed to be a change over of neighbours. Eva had gone and Sadie and Martha had appeared all bright eyed and bushy tailed for the day shift.

Nell had washed the baby's head and was drying his face with the soft towel when she noticed a strong resemblance to Charlie and she said, "Well Charlie you can't deny this one, he's your double!"

A sudden hush fell on the room and Nell knew instinctively that her slip of the tongue had put her foot right in it. Charlie was the neighbour. In fact, he was Eva's husband.

Quickly Nell said "…on the other hand maybe he is more like Winston

Churchill," and there were a few forced laughs from the day shift neighbours. Nell never allowed herself to make those kinds of remarks again. Instead she would say, "Who do you think he's like?"

Well, where was Mr. Blackie anyway? Charlie had certainly played the part of the devoted husband. It turned out that Bill Blackie was on an oil rig and was making his way home at that moment. No one had even mentioned him during that whole labour! Nell still thought the baby looked very much like Charlie but then, who knows? He may look like his dad too!

Everything complete, Nell buttoned her green double-breasted coat, slid the green belt through the green bakelite buckle and pulled to tighten it. She lifted the confinement case and headed for the door and on to another day.

Chapter 15
Clare Douglas

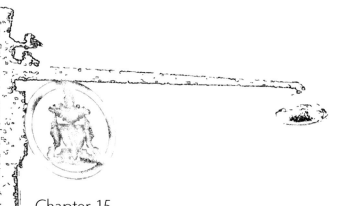

Clare Douglas hurried along Victoria Road toward her home in Pollokshields. She was walking at a fairly good pace, head down, unconsciously watching the patched concrete pavement as it passed beneath her; wee clumps of grass and the indestructible dandelions springing to life in cracks along the way. She had not planned on this pregnancy and had hoped to work more as a nurse at the Victoria Infirmary, when wee Ian was in school for the full day, come September. At the moment, he was only in school in the mornings. She wasn't unhappy about the pregnancy either; she loved her three boys, and they would manage fine. Clare had a good marriage with Ian, married twelve years! Mark was eleven, Dave was nine and wee Ian was five. Where has the time gone! They had hoped to sell their flat and buy a house with a garden in the suburbs, but that would probably have to wait another year. She was excited about the thought of her baby girl.

The segs on the heels of Clare's shoes made a clunk-click scraping noise on the concrete. It was almost hypnotizing. Deep in a dazed state she walked on, clunk-click like clockwork. She was thinking of her baby in her belly, baby Julie. She was due in three weeks time. The name had come easily, for July, the month of her birth. Clare knew that it was a girl. She secretly longed to dress a girl; pink frilly panties, angel tops, lacy tights and hats with bows and dancing classes. Her little girl in a pink and white fairy outfit on the stage being admired by everybody, then in skating lessons at Crossmyloof

Ice Rink. Clare had skated there as a child.

Julie's room would be like Shirley Temple's room with dancing shoes hanging on the wall and a big white teddy on her white organza girlie bed. Julie would have blue eyes, blonde curly hair and pink rose coloured cheeks. She would be the apple of her daddy's eye and her mother's pride and joy. Suddenly Clare was stopped in her tracks! Literally stopped by someone! Nell had come out of a close mouth and physically bumped into Clare!

"Steady on…Oh! Clare, it's you. You look as if you are miles away. How are you doing?" Nell's voice sang the last word in a higher pitch.

Clare stared at Nell for the longest time it seemed, then she burst into tears! Nell put her arm round Clare to steady and comfort her. They used to work in the same ward at the Southern General Hospital and Clare was one of Nell's booked cases for a home confinement.

"Lets head for that park bench just inside the gates there," said Nell motioning towards the gates of Queen's Park.

The two women sat down on the bench, unaware of the beautiful blooming purple rhododendron bush behind them. The bees were swarming in and out of the blossoms enjoying the June sunshine; they had to be busy when the sun was out as the Scottish weather was changeable and it could be snowing later in the day.

"Clare what's up?" asked Nell directly. Clare put her black, bucket bag down on the ground beside her and it tipped over. Out spilled bags with frilly baby clothes—there was a mass of pink and white at her feet.

"Oh Nell, I've not had any movement since last night!" sobbed Clare.

Nell fought back the usual clichés; *"You're kidding,"* or, *"Are you sure?"* "When did you last feel movement?" Nell asked determinedly.

"About seven o'clock last night. We were all sitting after our tea watching the Cilla Black show and all of a sudden I had this burst of movement. It was really strong; you could see it through my frock. It was intense and must have lasted about three or four minutes. Then there was nothing, not even a flicker or the occasional bump. She's never moved like that before. It struck me as strange, but I wasn't too worried till I got up this morning and got the boys ready for school and there wasn't the usual morning movement. When they left for school, I decided Julie and I should go shopping to buy clothes for her and maybe she would move."

As she spoke the tears rolled down Clare's cheeks. She licked them as they cascaded over her top lip, and still they came, but they did not ease the knife-like pain in her soul. She felt that the knife had impaled her to the park bench, right through her chest.

Nell hugged her as her tears convulsed into deep sobs. Nell did not want to give Clare any false hope. It was almost certain in Nell's mind that the baby had ceased to be alive. The frantic movement that Clare had described was the typical tragic description in so many of the stillbirths that Nell had witnessed.

"I'm going to get us a taxi to your place," said Nell, "and I'll check with the Pinnards and then call Dr. Mills."

"OK…OK," replied Clare between the sobs, as she pushed the back of her clenched hands into her reddened eyes in an attempt to well up the tears and compose herself. Her hands felt cool for an instant before they soaked up heat from her furnace eyes. Her eyes felt raw.

Nell bent down to pick up the spilled shopping. Amongst the assortment, Nell noticed a little pink and white musical clown lying face down on a beautiful white lace Christening gown in its cellulose packaging. They lay there on the dusty path…dashed hopes! Nell put the packages into the black bucket bag and a few bars of, *Slumber sweetly my dear*, issued forth from the little clown. The two women looked hard and long at each other and not a word was spoken.

Nell felt saddened and a sickening feeling gnawed at her stomach. She fought back the tears that wanted to flow in empathy, but she knew that a course of action was needed to carry Clare through this nightmare. Tears from Nell at that time would not have been helpful. The two women walked resolutely, arms linked, onto Victoria Road where Nell hailed a Black Hack taxicab. They sank into the sepulchral coolness of the black leather seats in the freshly cleaned cab.

"Where to hen?" asked the driver kindly, aware that all was not well with this hire.

"Kenmuir Street please, the far end, Driver," replied Nell.

"Righty oh," and the taxi gathered speed.

Home was the best place to face reality. Nell palpated Clare's abdomen and listened carefully with the Pinnards stethoscope. At one point her heart gave a leap. She counted a fast beat, 160 beats per minute exactly. She counted it over and over. She took Clare's pulse; 80 beats for a minute, exactly half of the 160. It was a uterine soufflé, and her heart sank into her boots again. She had heard the mother's pulse and an echo adding up to double the mother's pulse.

¤

Nell remembered as a student midwife she had recorded this as the foetal heart and felt so badly when she discovered that it was not the baby's heartbeat, but the uterine soufflé. There was no baby's heartbeat. The obstetrician kindly explained the phenomenon to Nell. In days gone by they used it as a tool to diagnose pregnancy. Thank goodness she had that piece of knowledge!

¤

"I cannot hear a heart beat, Clare," Nell said clearly.

"I know, I know, my poor wee mite, my wee Julie," said Clare looking at Nell. Her eyes were red and swollen and there were white streaks down her face from the dried salt of her tears.

"Do you want to contact Ian at work?" asked Nell.

"No Nell, he works at Chrysler in Linwood and it is a long drive home for him. I'll give the boys their lunch and wee Ian and I will go to the park. He loves to play on the paddleboats. We will pass the afternoon till Ian gets home at five. Nothing can be done now." Clare's saddened voice was composed, calm, and matter-of-fact.

"I'll phone Dr. Mills and get you an appointment for…say seven?"

"That will be fine Nell, and Ian will come with me to the doctor's surgery."

"Can you phone a friend or your mother?" asked Nell.

"I'd rather not, at the moment. I want Ian to know first and we will deal with the others afterwards."

"Good plan…Can I get you anything for the boy's lunch?" Nell offered.

"No, I have meat sauce in the fridge and I will boil up some spaghetti… they all love that so there won't be any hassle. They can have ice cream too."

"I'll see you tomorrow Clare. Have a good talk with Dr. Mills tonight."

"How long before I go into labour Nell?"

Nell dreaded that question because it could take up to three weeks before the doctor would induce Clare. The feeling was that if the mum was induced and the induction failed, then she would require a Caesarian Section for a dead baby, and that would be unacceptable. They would rather the labour was spontaneous. If it took as long as three weeks, then there was a risk to the mother of bleeding problems and infection. Some women hated the thought of the dead baby inside of them for days, but Clare had not expressed that feeling yet. Nell hoped that she would go into labour soon before the baby's skin began to peel.

"It may take a few days Clare. Talk it over with Dr. Mills."

"OK…I'll see you in the morning Nell…and thanks for picking up the pieces. I felt that I was going off my head."

"You were just trying to make sense of what was happening to you. You will get through this, Clare. If I get called out I'll phone you in the morning."

Nell fastened up her double breasted coat, slipped the green belt through the green bakelite buckle, tugged to tighten it then lifted her case and headed out. Nell walked along Kenmuir Street. It was relatively quiet and she was deep in thought planning the rest of her day.

She remembered one midwife saying to her when she became a Domiciliary Midwife, "You have to be flexible and take what comes."

It was true; Plan B was often carried out more than Plan A. It was almost lunch time, so Nell thought she would head for the Easy Eats Café for lunch, then catch up with the rest of her visits in the afternoon. She would phone the office too about Clare, in case Clare called the office. She had not wanted to use Clare's home phone and subject her to listening to her story over and over. Nell did not want a midwife to go there and not know that the baby was deceased.

The quiet was shattered, first by the school bell from Albert Drive School and second, by the roars of the children as they headed out of the school doors and home for lunch. Nell wondered why the children cheered as they left the building. However, looking back to her own childhood, she had done the same thing. "Hooray!" as she came out of the school doors.

It was freedom expressed! It was feeling expressed! How soon we curb our feelings into societal norms, Nell thought. She would love to scream at the top of her voice just now. She would love to shout, "It's not fair! It's not fair! Why? Why? Why?"

Nell watched the primary school children spill into the playground and then quickly go their own way home or to school dinners. She loved to watch the little groups form round some tidbit of interest. She watched four little girls look in turn into another's mouth, probably to see where the tooth had been.

Nell saw a bus coming her way in the distance and hurried to the bus stop. She was swamped with school children as she boarded and the clippie was shouting, "One at a time you lot! Ah hope, Sister, the weans that you bring grow up to be better behaved than this lot," and the clippie gave Nell a wink and a knowing nod. Nell soon alighted near the Easy Eats Café.

"Hello Sister, how's it gaun?" said Geoff as Nell swung the door of the Café open.

"Fair to middlin' Geoff."

"Oh wan o' they days? Never mind ye'll feel better efter a bite an' a wee cup o' tea."

"You're right there Geoff," said Nell: "I'll have a bacon and egg roll, a Tunnock's Caramel wafer and a pot of tea please."

"Coming right up Sister…. Bacon egg roll, pot of tea for the Sister," he called Nell's order to the back kitchen. It didn't take May long to bring the teapot, cup, saucer, teaspoon, knife and serviette.

"Here yi' are then Sister. Yir roll will jist be a wee minnit."

"Thanks May, how are the kids doing?" asked Nell.

"They are all fine Sister. In fact they baith huv their sports day this efternoon so Ah hope the weather stays dry."

"How's Roger doing with his running?"

"Aye fine Sister. He's been training hard wi' the Junior Bellahouston Harriers and the West of Scotland heats are next week." Geoff and May were both very proud of their son Roger, who just loved to run.

"It is wonderful that he has a hobby he is passionate about," said Nell.

"Aye weel it keeps him oot o' mischief an tae tell yi the truth, it's good fur him jist noo as he's been bullied a bit at school; but he wins nearly aw the sports awards so that puts the bully's gas in a peep!"

Another example of a typical Glasgow expression, Nell thought.

"Here yi' are noo, wan roll wi' egg an' Ayrshire bacon. Enjoy…" May smiled as she served Nell.

"Thanks May…and how are Crystal and wee Jim?"

"She will have her highland dancing display next week, and Jim is dain fine. I think he will be a runner too…he likes to run efter Roger!"

"Fun an' games, eh?"

"Yir no kiddin' Sister! They say it keeps yi young but Ah don't know about that…doesnae feel like that," said May with a big grin on her face. She just loved her kids.

Nell, in turn, loved the smell and taste of Ayrshire bacon. She would savour it. She stirred her tea in the "Tree of India" patterned cup and took a sip…yes, the cup that cheers…a wee cup of tea to sooth the troubled soul.

The next morning found Nell standing in Clare's kitchen mixing some bicarbonate of soda with a large dose of castor oil and fresh orange juice.

"Try and drink it while it is frothing," Nell said as she handed the tumbler to Clare.

Dr. Mills had ordered an OBE. Not an Order of the British Empire medal but Oil, Bath and Enema. This was called a medical induction, as opposed to the surgical induction, which was rupturing the membranes (breaking the waters). The idea behind the medical induction was, as Nell understood, the castor oil would cause stimulation of the bowel and the rectum that lay next to the birth canal and hopefully it would stimulate the cervix to release prostaglandin, which is a hormone found inside the neck of the womb. Then the bath would cause an increase in blood supply to the area and the enema would cause a mass emptying of the rectum and lower bowel.

Hopefully, in all of the rumblings and tumult of the proceedings, the cervix would be stimulated and the mother would go full steam ahead into labour. It sometimes worked if the woman was about to go into labour anyway and the cervix was ripe (soft). One drawback was that the castor oil had a habit of repeating over and over and over again throughout the labour. Nell prayed that it would work in Clare's case. Clare had opted to stay at home instead of going into hospital. She also wanted an undertaker to deal with the baby and have a proper burial.

There was an option at that time for the hospital to cremate the stillbirth. It was felt it would be less traumatic to the mum and family if it was taken out of their hands. There was no charge for the service.

Later that evening, the call came. "It's Ian Douglas here. Clare said could you come now Nell?"

"I'll be along soon Ian," said Nell.

Nell phoned straight away for a car and the gas and air machine. A student nurse would be attending the birth too, if Clare did not mind. Nell requested that the student should come in the same car so that she could brief her on the situation and negate the asking of many questions. After all, this was now about Clare and Ian.

Nell was pleased to see Bette Fairly, the student midwife, sitting in the car when it arrived to fetch her. This will be OK, thought Nell.

Nell filled Bette in with Clare's story. "Have you seen a stillbirth before Bette?" asked Nell.

"Yes," Bette replied, "but the baby was a wee thing of thirty weeks gestation. They wondered too if it was really only about twenty-seven weeks."

These cases were difficult as twenty-eight weeks was the legal cut off point for viability; under twenty eight weeks the foetus was considered an abortion.

"This will be so different then. This baby is just over thirty-six weeks gestation and probably about six to seven pounds in weight." Nell tried to prepare Bette as best she could.

"It is so sad, Sister, to have carried a baby that long and then to have an intrauterine death," said Bette perplexed.

"There is one thing that I should mention to you. Everything is very quiet and still when the baby is born, so don't feel that you have to speak to keep the conversation going. Conversation will flow if Clare and Ian want that. We will let them lead the way," Nell advised.

"Do we know why the baby died?" asked Bette.

"Good question Bette. I spoke with Dr. Mills about that very thing and we have looked over the prenatal record, but there are no hints there. There was no gestational diabetes or apparent infection. It could be viral, though or the cord round the baby's neck or a true knot in the cord. When the membranes rupture there will probably be thick meconium; the bowels always move if there is distress. From the history I think that this baby had been in distress."

"The stillbirth that I saw in hospital," Bette recalled, "the mother was a diabetic."

"Yes, they have a tough time carrying their babies past thirty-five weeks," Nell explained " Oh here we are…"

Nell and Bette got out of the car. Bette picked up the gas and air machine. They headed to the second floor, to the Douglas' home. It was ten thirty in the evening. Clare was definitely in labour and the contractions were giving her some grief. Nell examined Clare and found the cervix to be three finger breadths dilated.

"Clare you do not have to suffer anymore pain," Nell advised.

"OK Nell, but I talk nonsense when I have pethidine," said Clare.

"Well we have been warned about the nonsense," smiled Nell, "…now for the injection."

"Oh! I nearly forgot!" said Clare, "Dr. Mills gave me a prescription for morphine vials…it's on the chest of drawers over there beside that bottle of nail varnish."

It always interested Nell where patients kept dangerous drugs such as morphine and pethidine. The Dangerous Drug Act demanded that they be kept in a locked cupboard within a cupboard and be counted every shift change and each dose signed for in the hospital situation. In the home situation, Nell found them in the strangest places. When she was doing General District Nursing, one lady told her that the pethidine pills were beside the cat's fish and the firelighters on the kitchen windowsill!

Clare had her morphine injection. There was no need to worry about the drug reaching the baby in this case. The morphine gave an air of well being to Clare so she chatted easily to Ian who had been struggling with the situation. This helped him cope. He saw her relaxed. Nell timed the contractions, but it was strange not to have to keep checking the foetal heart. Clare was progressing well in labour. The hours passed with occasional chat.

"I told the boys tonight about the baby. I don't think that they really understood. They were very quiet," said Clare.

"Oh, I think they understood more than you think Clare. I heard Mark and Dave talking about it and they decided that they won't cry in front of you as it would make you 'ore sad," Ian said.

"Oh Ian! The wee souls. We'll talk it out with them after…"

"Yes we will have a lot of talking to do I dare say…are you feeling any pain?" asked Ian looking at Clare's face grimace.

"No not really but I am beginning to feel pressure down below. Do you think that I could be ready to push Nell?"

"Let's have a look then…. There is a bit of bulging…I think that your waters are about to go…yes…you will feel less pressure for a bit…"

Thick meconium stained fluid drained on to the pads that Nell had placed on the bed. Nell checked Clare.

"You are ready to push when you feel like doing so Clare. Just wait till you feel that pressure build up," suggested Nell.

There was a Grandmother clock on the fireplace wall that kept a steady tick. Nell had not noticed it until then. Now that the talking had ceased, the clock's pendulum was a focal point.

"Nell I'm pushing and I can't help it," grunted Clare.

"That's fine. Just do what your body tells you to do. Easy does it Clare…"

Clare pushed while the pendulum didn't miss a swing. Thirty minutes swung away before Julie Douglas was born, stillborn, at three 3:14 a.m. Clare was right, it was a wee girl. All was still…even the clock seemed to hush its relentless tick-tock, as their senses were filled with emotion. The air was charged with solemn-ness.

"Julia, I will wrap you up and give you to your mum and dad…they want to hold you." Nell's voice was soft and calm hiding the gut wrench that she was experiencing.

"Come on ma' wee thing," said Clare as Ian put his arms round both of them.

Tears cascaded over the little still cherub in their arms. Bette and Nell worked quietly to deliver the afterbirth and complete the confinement. They found a true knot in the cord, which had been pulled tight and cut off the baby's oxygen supply. Why? Why? Why? There was nothing that anyone could have done to prevent this.

They left the trio and went into the other room to do all their charting. After about ten minutes they heard two strained crackling voices singing,

> *Safe in the arms of Jesus*
> *Safe on his gentle breast*
> *There by his love o'ershaded*
> *Sweetly her soul shall rest.*

Bette wept. Nell patted her shoulder with one hand and wiped the tears away from her own eyes with the other. Clare asked Nell to dress Julia in her Christening robe and hat before she left. This she did and placed Julia on a soft feather pillow. The boys would see her before the undertaker would come for her. Nell was relieved that the baby's face was intact. The little blue life-less face, in the white lacy outfit, would haunt Nell for days. Bette and Nell prepared to leave the Douglas Family.

Nell buttoned her double-breasted coat, slipped the green belt through the bakelite buckle and tugged to tighten it. She lifted her case and headed out.

¤

Nell and Bette attended the funeral of Julie Douglas. It was a tearful ceremony for all that attended. The Douglas family moved to Clarkston shortly afterwards and wee Ian went to school for the full day in September. Clare eventually returned to work, after Christmas.

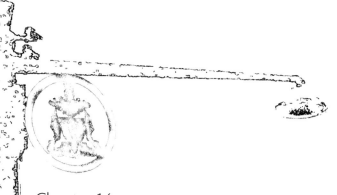

Chapter 16
Annie Shaw

"Hello…Annie?…Annie Shaw…? Oh! I'm Sister Dickson the midwife…Sister McGilvery's on holiday just now," said Nell as Annie appeared in the opened doorway.

This was a top floor tenement flat in Norfork St. in Gorbals, just a few streets away from the River Clyde, and the noise of the heavy diesel traffic seemed to get louder, the higher Nell climbed. It was a warm day and the heat in the stairwell rose with each step. Nell was pleased to move up from the strong urine smell of the close. These closes were at ground level near to the bus routes and were often used as public toilets by men on their way home at night from the public houses. The ground floor flats were usually converted into businesses, so there were no tenants at that level to keep an eye on things.

It was hot and the air was still. Nell was thankful that she had left her coat at home and wore a fine green cardigan over her green uniform dress.

"Oh come on in Sister…Ye'll be fair wabbit efter they stairs, they dae me in tae…come away in the hoose…We're aw through in ra kitchen."

Annie had all the windows open to cool the place down and the through draughts were a welcome relief as Nell entered the cool hallway of the spacious tenement flat. Annie was expecting her fourth baby and Nell was making the booking visit today.

Nell followed Annie through the hallway to the far end where she entered a big bright kitchen, which was floored with orange and brown patterned inlaid linoleum. The kitchen had the old-fashioned black iron coal fire range complete with the "wally dugs" looking at each other across the mantelpiece. In the fireplace below a kettle was boiling merrily away on the hob and a light odour of curry rose from a large pot beside it. The room appeared uncluttered and sparkling clean. There were two fireside chairs, a solid oak table with six chunky dining chairs, a sideboard and a couple of occasional chairs with wicker backs. The two large pulleys, which spanned the ceiling, easily supported the family's laundry.

"Have a seat. A wee cuppa' char Sister?"

"That would be nice, weak with no milk or sugar, thanks Annie," Nell said as she took her cardigan off and draped it over a chair at the table. Then she brought out the paperwork that she needed and placed that on the table. It was good to sit down, as she had walked along Eglinton Street and Bridge Street for quite some way.

"Hello everyone," said Nell as she looked around the room. "I'm Sister Dickson…my it's a hot day and it's only ten o'clock!"

Nell nodded to the assembled women. There was a rather stout pleasant woman in a blue and white floral cotton frock. She sat at the open window, which had a cushion on its sill in readiness for "hingin'oot" over the back court. The frock had a white seersucker collar, which showcased an array of chins. It was buttoned to just below the waist round where a white patterned plastic belt fastened with an ornate buckle.

The woman was idly playing with her white "pop-it" plastic necklace beads. Her hair was graying and she had it up in rolls; one round the back of her hair head from ear to ear, and the second, a glamorous larger roll sweeping the bulk of her hair on top of her head. The total coiffeur was crowned with a black harness hairnet lest any wisp of hair escape. She wore large hoop gypsy earrings. Her bare legs, complete with matching bulging varicose veins, were terminally encased in a pair of well worn whitish sandals, the cross-wise straps of which trussed the tops of the feet like two rolls of pale, pork pot roast reminiscent of a butcher's weekend window. In all she was dressed for the weather!

"Aye hen it is hoat," said Kathy in the blue and white frock, replying to Nell's comment on the weather.

"It's gonna be a scorcher, aye! As sure as Goad's in Govan ye'll roast the day." Kathy was Annie's mother.

The other occupants of the room were three younger women in their twenties, Nell guessed. There was a hard looking wee nut, Senga, with peroxide blonde hair, a black brocade mini-skirt and a putrid pink low-necked top, which decorated, rather than covered, her buxom bosom. Senga, Nell gathered, was Annie's lodger, and she flapped about in her bare feet in and out of the room, obviously getting ready for something special.

The other two were neighbours, Big Isa and Wee Trish, who were in for a morning cup of tea and a smoke. Woodbine smoke wafted its way to the open window where Kathy would give the occasional cough and fan of the hand in displeasure as a trail of smoke lazily looped towards her.

"Ah don't mind folk smokin' but Ah don't waant it up ma nose," protested Kathy.

"Well don't sit there Ma," said Annie to her mother in a matter of fact way.

"Ah sit here fur the wee breeze as Ah wis bile-in' efter climbing they sters o' yours. Auch Ah'll jist get awa doon tae the butcher's shoap an get ma mince fur the night an' whit can Ah git you, hen?" asked Kathy

"A pun o' beef links fur the weans's tea Ma, cos they don't like that vegetable curry that Jazz is makin'…an' you drink a gless o' watter afore ye go, Ah don't want ye tae dehydrate."

"Naw. Ah don't need a drink the noo hen, it'll huv tae be hoatter than this tae turn me intae a prune. Ah'll see ye later. Cheerio Sister an tell her tae take mair rest wull ye?" pointing at Annie.

Kathy then turned to Big Isa and Wee Trish. "Come oan you yins…drink up an get movin' an let the Sister dae whit she hus tae dae."

Now that she had sorted everyone out, Kathy trundled out of the room with her navy blue message bag swinging over her right arm and her accordion purse held in the tight grip of her right hand.

As she passed through the hallway she was heard to say, "Ah hope yir' cleanin' up efter yirsel Senga, an' no leavin' it tae ma Annie. Remember her condition noo…" Then in a quieter voice, "Guid luck th'day hen at ra' clinic."

"She's a right bossy boots yoor Ma," said Big Isa, laughing.

"She is that Isa…but her hert's in the right place…I often wonder what keeps her goin' efter aw that she's been through. She came here this mornin' tae see the kids afore they went on their picnic to Rouken Glen."

"Is that where they're away tae?" asked Big Isa. "I wondered where they were gawin'. Ah saw aboot ten weans waitin' at the tram stoap."

"Aye that wid be them an' ma mammy broat packets o' crisps an' the like fur them an' gied them money fur ice cream and ra' boats."

"Awe! She his goat a hert o' gold the ole soul…Ah used tae like ra' oary boats masel at Rouken Glen. That's where Ah met Erchie MacCracken…mind him?" Asked Big Isa.

"It wis mair than his name that wis cracken if Ah'm thinkin' oan the right wan…That wis him ye went tae Blackpool wi' fur the illuminations…wis it?" asked Annie.

"Aye that wis him awe right," replied Big Isa "…Ah thought that he wis ma knight in shinin' armour…but he and his hoarse bolted when he thought Ah wis pregnant an' Ah never saw hide nor hair o' him again."

"Were you pregnant Isa?" asked Wee Trish, who had been listening intently while balancing about an inch of cigarette ash on the remaining stump of the woodbine she was smoking.

"Naw Ah wisnae Trish…but he wis ma first boyfriend. It wis nice while it lasted but there was such a stramash at Rouken Glen that time cos he took the oars aff us lassies an we were floatin' about an' bangin' intae they islands in the middle o' ra watter. The Parkie wis fair fummin' at him…we awe thought it wis rare fun then. Aye…gone are ra' days…Oh here! Ah better go an get ma messengers afore it gets too stifling…cumoan Trish, Ah'll walk yi doon ra road hen." 'Messages' was a common Glasgow term for groceries but many Glasgow folk called them 'messengers'.

"Aye, Ah better get ma erse in gear too," said Wee Trish carefully depositing the cigarette end complete with the column of ash in the fire.

"Ta ta ra noo then Annie. Thanks for the tea. Ah'll see you later hen…Cheerio Sister." And off they went like Mutt and Geoff, the long and short of things to come.

Nell gave them a wave as they departed. Big Isa called to Senga as they left, "Hope yi get the aw' clear at the clinic Senga. We'll probably see yi later."

That left Annie in the kitchen and Senga was still flapping about in the other part of the house performing ablutions of sorts by the diverse noises that were heard.

"Senga hus tae go back tae Black Street Clinic the day. She's a wee bit nervy aboot it," explained Annie.

Black Street Clinic housed the Venereal Disease Clinic. The Goddess Venus has a lot to answer for; venereal disease being one! Not many of the sufferers care about where the name came from—Venus the Goddess of

Love.

"You're not afraid of her living here in such close proximity with you and your children?" Nell asked in a concerned voice.

"Naw Sister there's nothin' tae worry boot…it's no VD is only Gonorrhea!"

Nell smiled a wry smile at Annie and thought, where ignorance is bliss 'tis folly to be wise. The dreaded Venereal Disease was Syphilis!

"Gonorrhea is still serious, Annie, it falls under Venereal diseases too you know;" Nell informed Annie.

"Aye, but Ah think she's clear noo an' she's been away tae see hir mammy in Port Glesga' awe week as she could'nae work oan ra' game till she goat the aw' clear frae ra' clinic."

"You have a busy time of it in the mornings, Annie. Do they all visit you every morning?"

"Aye, maist mornings if Jazz is workin. You see Sister, they're aw a bit lost oan their ain so they congregate here in the mornings.…Ah really don't mind as Ah worry aboot Isa and Trish if Ah don't see them…an' ma mammy's on hir own so Ah wid huv tae go doon there tae see she's OK."

Annie's mother, Kathy, was widowed when Annie's father was killed in action in 1944. He was in the Black Watch Regiment. Annie pointed to a tall smart kilted man in a brownish photograph that had pride of place on the mantelpiece. Kathy never remarried, but brought up five kids on a war pension and washed tenement stairs four days a week.

The tenement stairs had to be cleaned by the tenants who took their turn of sweeping and washing them once a week…from their landing to the landing below. Tenants on the ground floor did the front close and close mouth and the back close. Many people hired a "Mrs. Mop" to do this chore. They were often called the "stair wummin". If someone lost their job or was short of money a common phrase was, "I'll need tae take in stairs to wash."

Kathy had been a Mrs. Mop. She had her own clientele and in a way, had her own tax free business. She always had ready cash and this eked out her pension money so her children never went without. She was always there when they came home from school. She kept tabs on her boys, in case they would get into trouble, but they did not give her too much hassle.

Annie's three brothers immigrated to America to the Detroit area to work in the car industry. They still kept in touch with Kathy and she had been to see them in Detroit with all expenses paid. She was proud of them. Annie's sister Joan met an American sailor who was stationed at the Polaris Submarine Base in the Holy Loch. They were married in Glasgow and she immigrated to Texas, where they had to be married (to each other) again. Kathy's comment on the double wedding was; "It's a load o' tripe. They Yanks don't know their erse frae their elbow."

However, Joan wrote to Kathy every month and came back to Glasgow periodically to see her. When she did, she usually took Kathy away on holiday. Joan did not have any children, but all of her brothers did. So there was just Annie in Glasgow and Ruby who had stayed with the family since 1947 when she was orphaned. The authorities would not let Kathy legally adopt Ruby because of her circumstances, but Ruby wanted to live with Kathy, so the powers that be allowed a long term fostering arrangement.

Ruby's mother and Kathy had been best pals since school days. Ruby was an only child and just adored Kathy. Ruby, now married and living in Shawlands, made sure that she saw Kathy at least once every week. Over the years Kathy had accepted Annie's relationship with Jazz, who was a seaman from Calcutta. Kathy liked Jazz Singh, and called him the 'gentle giant'. He was a quiet kindly gentleman of six feet two inches in his bare feet.

Kathy loved her grandchildren and got upset when they were called names because of their mixed color. "Half-caste" was a term used to describe someone who had one Indian and one Scottish parent. Kathy was determined that they would do well at school and tried to encourage them in their studies. She did want them to a get good job like Ruby; just with a wee bit hard work Ruby got a start in the Clydesdale Bank and had done well for herself. Kathy considered herself lucky. She was proud of her family and she had her own small tenement flat. She had good neighbours and friends, and did not owe a penny to anybody. She had a reason to get up in the morning.

Big Isa was twenty-eight and had known Annie for about twelve years. Isa was five feet nine with a slim figure and jet black long hair. She had worked with Annie in the same pub, the Oxford Arms, as a barmaid. In fact, Annie was instrumental in getting Isa a job there.

This pub was busy and was near the docks, so it was usually frequented with sailors and dockers. It tended to be a bit rough and tumble sort of place. When Isa first got the job she was living in a derelict building with a couple of boys. There was nothing romantic between them they were just trying to survive from day to day; the three of them had run away from home the same day.

Isa had lived in Drumchapel and her father had abused her both sexually and physically until she couldn't stand it any longer. When she found out that her mother knew what was happening and didn't do anything to stop it, she packed up and left. Her parents never tried to find her. The abuse had started when Isa was about nine. Every Tuesday night her mother would go to Bridgeton from Drumchapel to visit Isa's Gran and she did not get back till the eleven o'clock bus. Isa had to see that her young brother and sister would get to bed about eight o'clock.

Isa's father went to his bed early to read the paper and listen to his radio. At nine o'clock, he banged on the floor with his size ten work boot and Isa had to take him up a cup of Horlicks and two digestive biscuits. That went on for some time, then he would order her to undress naked and parade up and down in front of him. She hated doing this and tried various ploys to avoid it. She cried, but that seemed to goad him on to make her pose in different positions. She ignored him and would not look in his direction but that made him angry. She scowled at him and that seemed to have some effect by making the session shorter.

When her Gran died, Isa heaved a sigh of relief; she felt guilty about feeling pleased that her mother would not have to go out on a Tuesday night. To Isa's utter dismay, her mother still went out on a Tuesday night. Isa didn't know that her father made her mother go out.

The abuse became more invasive as Isa developed and matured into a young woman. He would make her stand near the bed and he would fondle her breasts and genitalia. He told her if she said anything to her mother he would do the same to her wee sister and he would scar her face so badly that she would not want anyone to see her. She believed him. Her father was a big man with a heavy dark growth and he began to expose himself to her and make her lie down beside him. He would push his penis into her mouth, which made her boak. Then he finally forced her to have intercourse with him. She hated it and hated him. She wanted to kill him and she could not stand it anymore.

Finally she told her mother! Her mother knew all along as he had been threatening her that he would sexually abuse the younger sister too. Isa left that next Tuesday afternoon.

Isa met the two lads, Keith and Bruce, on her first night away from home when she was looking for somewhere to sleep. They had come up from Greenock on the train and the three of them sneaked into Central station and slept in parked train carriages. They did not get much sleep, but at least it was dry and relatively safe. They looked out for one another and they slept on the trains for a few nights till the train they were in was shunted to a junction near Pollokshields Station. They managed to get out of the mass of railway lines and made it safely onto Eglinton Street.

Some of the buildings in the Gorbals were condemned, and they found a place to live as squatters. It was then that Isa met Annie, when she was trailing all the pubs and shops looking for work. Annie took Isa in till she saved enough money for a place she shared with another girl. Annie was able to give Keith and Bruce the name of a coal merchant in the Gorbals so they could get some work.

Isa never went back to Drumchapel. Even if she saw a bus with "Drumchapel" on the front of it, her heart would miss a beat and she would get all sweaty and her throat would dry up. She never ate digestive biscuits again nor would she have Horlicks in the house. She had been greatly traumatized and Annie had been a faithful friend to her.

Keith and Bruce became good friends to Isa; they were like brothers to her. All three had had to endure the trauma of dysfunctional families and they had a lot of emotional baggage to shed. They had all been robbed of their innocence and part of their childhood. It took Isa a long time to even look at a boy and that had been Archie McCracken in the Rouken Glen episode.

Isa was now married to Phil, who worked in the bookie's office and they had one daughter Jess, who was five. They would not have any more children, as Isa had a hysterectomy just after Jess was born because half of the placenta was attached into the muscle of the womb and she was bleeding profusely. To save her life, the flying squad had to be called and the Obstetrician at Rotten Row had to perform an emergency hysterectomy for partial placenta accreta. Nell had heard of this case and was pleased that Isa looked so well. She and Phil had a happy life together and Jess was well loved.

Isa and Phil lived across the landing from Phil's mother and father so she had a built-in baby sitter. Isa still worked as a barmaid in the same pub. It was in the Oxford Arms that she had first experienced friendship, warmth, and comfort. She always felt safe there, for the first time in her saddened young life.

Annie first met Wee Trish when Trish was about nine, when she first was called to walk her mother home from the pub. Trish would come faithfully every night and take her drunken mother home when the pub closed. It was sad to see this happen night after night. Both Trish's mother and father were alcoholics and it was impossible to see any betterment for any of them. It hadn't always been that way. Till the age of nine, Trish had enjoyed a happy childhood. She stayed with her parents and her Granny. Her Granny was her mother's mother. "The Granny you canny shove off the bus," Trish always said.

Her father, Roger, was in the Royal Navy and she remembered him always being very handsome in his naval uniform. When he left the navy he worked in the Clydeside shipyards. He did not settle on land and often said he hadn't found his land legs yet. But life was not so bad, even after her Granny died and there was just the three of them.

Trish's mother, Jan, had been brought up strict Brethren; no dancing or drinking or going to the pictures was allowed. Times changed and she began to do all of these things more and more with Roger, since her mother was no longer there to point the finger. She would just have a wee gin and orange when they went out, and then another when they got back and so on and so on. The wee gin and orange was Trish's mother's ruin. For the longest time Trish thought that her mother was drinking orange juice. Jan had a drinking problem and Roger tried to help her out, but soon he was part of a double drinking problem.

Trish had been a good student at school and she had wanted to stay on till fifth year to do her highers, but money was tight and she left school at fifteen with her Third Year Leaving Certificate in all subjects. She did get a job in the pharmacy section of Boots the Chemists, at the corner of Argyll Street and Renfield Street, commonly known as Boots' Corner. She had no life of her own, trying to cope with two alcoholics. Her father managed to work and hold on to his job, but her mother was fired from her office job as she was found "tippling in the loo".

It was Isa who finally helped Trish to leave her parents and move out and have a life of her own. Isa took Trish to an Al-a-non meeting, which was held in Queen Street near Queen Street Station. Trish had burst into tears when she heard the familiar stories and realized she was not to blame for her parent's drinking. She stopped facilitating their lifestyle and moved out. She got new job in a department store in Argyle Street in the hat department, and began to have friends of her own and a life away from her parents. When she started going out with a group to a cocktail bar she would order a bloody Mary just because she had once heard a rather sophisticated lady ordering this. She soon found that she had the same problem as her parents and hit the bottle hard.

It was Isa again, who then took her to an AA meeting and Trish straightened herself out with the twelve-step program. She hadn't married and now worked with Isa in the Pub. Trish claimed if she worked with booze she would not want to drink it, however she had fallen off the wagon from time to time. Trish went to AA every week to keep her in sobriety. She had a framed copy of the Serenity Prayer in the pub and at home.

The Serenity Prayer

God grant me the serenity
To accept the things I cannot change…
Courage to change the things that I can…
And the wisdom to know the difference…

Trish had to put the sentiments in this prayer into action when she was called out in the middle of the night when her parents set their bed on fire. Both were in a drunken state and both died of smoke inhalation.

She, of course, blamed herself for their deaths, even though the firemen told her that she would have certainly died too if she had been sleeping in the house. Annie and Isa were both her sounding boards and safety net. Even Kathy would visit her in those tough days after the fire.

Trish had had many boyfriends but she always said, "He's too fond o' ra bevy fur me. Ah'll need a teetotaller…an that's hard to find in Glasgow especially in a Pub! Ah might need tae go tae ra' Band o' Hope!"

Annie and Isa always told her that Mr. Right would come along one day.

Trish's reply was always the same. "When ma ship comes in, knowin' ma luck A'll be waitin' at Dundas Street bus Station!"

This was the cue for them to laugh, but there was a sadness in the laughter, for Trish hadn't had much luck to date.

Nell finally got all the booking history taken from Annie. Annie was a kindly person, quietly strong in character and was happy with her lot in life. She did not have any ambition to move away from the Gorbals. She knew where she was and was content with that. She was one of the first

Caucasian patients that Nell had met whose common law husband was an Indian man. Annie did, however, have ambitions for her children. She was the constant in so many lives that surrounded her.

Nell put the paperwork back in the lining of her case and arranged to visit Annie again before Sister McGilvery came back. Annie's blood pressure was on the border line of high so Nell did tell her to take a rest every afternoon, "not just because your mother told me to," she laughed with Annie.

"Aye Sister A'll dae that, Jazz is a great help and he does maist o' ra cookin' fur me. I hope ye meet him the next time ye call."

"I hope so too," said Nell as she put the baumanometer and the urine testing equipment in her case and fastened the case and the cover. She said her goodbyes to Annie and left with a wealth of feeling for Annie and Annie's circle of friends.

It had only been thirty minutes…as she passed through the hallway she called to Senga, "Hope things go well for you at Black Street today."

"Ta Sister," shouted Senga in return.

Nell slipped on her fine green cardigan, over her green uniform, lifted her case, and set off into the warm summer's day.

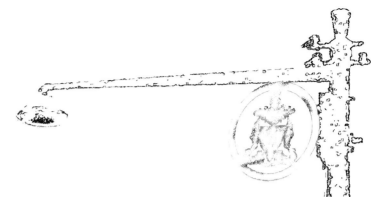

Chapter 17
Nosey Rosey

The phone was ringing as Nell put the key in her door. She quickly lifted the receiver and answered with the number. "You sound out of puff sister," said Miss Wilson.

"Oh I'm just in the door Miss Wilson," said Nell.

"Well there is a B.B.A. (Born Before Arrival) in your area in Netherlee, so call a taxi and then call me back for the details."

"Will do," Nell replied. She called the nearest taxi rank, then the office to get the correct address and the patient's name. Everything was a bit hazy, as the neighbour who phoned did not know much about the situation. The address was in a terrace house in Netherlee. It was in a very quiet street and the woman had just recently moved to the area.

Nell arrived at the Reid's home. A neighbour, Rose McPherson, answered the door and showed Nell upstairs into the front bedroom. Sylvia was sitting up in bed drinking the last of a big mug of hot cream of tomato soup Rose had brought in for her. Nell could hear Rose downstairs feeding the other two children in the kitchen. The baby was tucked in beside Sylvia at her left side. Nell felt the baby's cheek and neck and realized that it was cool to touch, so she didn't waste any time in setting to work.

Nell drew back the covers and found that the baby, wrapped in a damp towel, was still attached to the placenta, which was situated between Sylvia's legs in a pool of congealed blood. Nell cut the cord and quickly dried and wrapped the baby in a dry, warm towel. Rose had put on the gas fire and laid some things out for Nell to bath the baby.

The baby's temperature was 95.8 degrees, which was too low for a bath. Nell called to Rose for a hot water bottle. Rose brought up two new filled rubber hot water bottles, which had fleecy buttoned covers on them. Nell rubbed the baby dry and dressed him in a hat, mitts, bootees and nappy and swaddled him in fine warmed flannelette baby sheets. Then she wrapped him in a baby blanket and put him in his carry cot and placed one hot water bottle below him and one at his back; he was lying on his right side. Over all this she placed a down quilt.

She knew that she would have to get the baby to feed, but while he was heating up she examined Sylvia and helped her out of the mess she was in. She gathered the placenta into an asher (dish) that had been put aside for this purpose. The placenta looked complete; she would examine it later as at present there were more urgent things to do. Sylvia's condition was stable, so that was a big plus. Nell quickly changed Sylvia's bed and cleaned up the mess.

As the story unfolded, Nell discovered that it was Sylvia Reid's third child, a brother for Anne and John who were 5 years and 3 years old, respectively. Her husband, Craig, was a policeman who has just been transferred to this Glasgow detachment from Edinburgh. They moved into the house only three days earlier and had only briefly met a couple of the neighbours. Craig was away on a training course all week. The baby was not due for another three weeks. Sylvia and Craig's family all lived in the Edinburgh area, so she was on her own.

"There you are Sylvia you are on dry land once again," smiled Nell.

"That feels warmer already sister, I didn't know what to do when the afterbirth came away just after I got into bed."

"You did the right thing Sylvia," Nell reassured her, "The baby is a wee bit colder that I would want for him, but we will get him warmed up."

Nell lifted the baby and put one of the hot water bottles into the bed. The other she left in the carry cot. The baby was still fast asleep but did feel a bit warmer now; his temperature had increased. She tried to waken the baby and encouraged Sylvia to put the baby in her cleavage for heat and the proximity to the breast might waken him. Sylvia was going to breastfeed, as she had done so with her other children. As she attempted to feed the baby, she expressed some colostrums (which is very sweet) onto the baby's lips and tongue. The baby showed little interest and slept on.

"Keep cuddling him Sylvia and keep him warm. I'm going downstairs to make up some sugar and water for him," said Nell.

"OK Sister he feels a bit warmer already, there we are mum's big boy… just you wait till your daddy sees you!"

Sylvia reclined back on the pillows and cuddled her new son. She sang a verse of *Dream Angus* to him as she rocked him from side to side.

"*…hush now my bairn and sleep without greeting, dream Angus will bring you a dream my dear…*"

Nell was thinking they needed a march, not a lullaby to wake this baby up, but it was good to see mother and baby bonding. Nell prepared an ounce of sugar and boiled water and tried to feed the baby with a teaspoon; no luck. Nell checked the baby's temperature. It had improved a little 96.4. Nell did not like this. It had struck her at the first glance that the baby's head had excessive moulding. He looked like a cone head. She asked Rose, who had a phone in her home, to call Dr. Moore.

Nell tried to piece the story together. For moulding like that to occur on the baby's head, Sylvia would have been in labour for a lengthy time, so why was she a B.B.A.?'

The pieces of this puzzle began to emerge when Sylvia explained, "You see Sister I didn't have the front contractions that I had with the other two."

"Every labour is different Sylvia but yes, you usually have the front contractions," replied Nell.

"I did have back pain but I thought that I had aggravated an old back injury by unpacking some of the packing cases. I did try to be careful," continued Sylvia.

"Did you have any show?" asked Nell.

"No not really," replied Sylvia, "I just had the start of a cold."

"Your throat does sound a bit croaky," Nell commented.

"My plan was to go for Anne's appointment to be registered at school, get a few groceries and lie on the couch, rest my back and read the kids some stories. Craig had made me promise that I would take it easy today. He said that I had done too much yesterday."

"That sounded like a good plan, but you know what Rabbie said, "The best laid plans o'mice and men gang aft aglay." Nell smiled.

"Luckily I had taken the go-chair with me, as wee John gets tired sometimes. I needed it to lean on as my back was killing me, especially on the way back. I thought I was going to go through the go-chair," Sylvia grimaced.

"You poor girl, you were probably in the second stage of labour then. You could have had the baby in the street!" Nell exclaimed.

"When I stepped into the house I felt sick as if I was going to have diarrhea, so I gave the children a drink and a packet of biscuits each (something that I never do) and I switched on the TV for their programme and rushed to the toilet."

"You must have been experiencing involuntary pushing," Nell followed.

"I was absolutely flabbergasted when the baby plopped into the toilet bowl. I quickly fished him out and I saw he was breathing. I wrapped him in a towel then felt all clammy and dizzy…I remember holding onto the edge of the bath with one hand and holding the baby close to me with the other…then I must have fainted."

"It was fortunate that you held the baby to you as you slumped to the floor. What an ordeal for you," Nell empathized.

"When I came to I had my arms round the baby and I heard banging on the door. It was Rose. Luckily the door wasn't locked and I called for her to come in. Rose had seen the children walking along the inside window-sill and wondered if I knew what they were doing."

"About what time would you say this happened?" asked Nell.

"I have no idea," replied Sylvia, "but the Ice Cream Man was playing his little tune in the street. I think that's why the children would have gone to the window."

"Well I'll phone the company and we will get a time of birth for the notification of birth form. Rose can perhaps give us an idea of the time frame too," suggested Nell.

"Rose helped me up the stairs into bed. I sat on every stair and that's how we did it and then the afterbirth came away when I got into bed. This is a new mattress. Thank goodness I left the plastic on it for the confinement or it would be ruined," Sylvia smoothed her hand over the bedclothes.

Nell tried feeding the baby again, but he would open his eyes briefly and then flop again into a sleep. His temperature was a bit better, but Nell was still worried. In the hospital nursery, she had once before seen this excessive moulding on a baby girl who had a tentorial tear (a membrane in the brain) and she died. This baby's sleepiness reminded Nell of that little baby girl. It could just be the cold injury, but the baby needed calories, as his blood sugar was probably used up by trying to keep as warm as he could; he was probably using up his brown fat stores at present.

Rose McPherson was the local busy body. She was always at her window and saw everything that happened in the neighbourhood. Her nickname was "Nosey Rosey" and Nell knew of her from a confinement she had in this area last year. One thing about Nosey Rosey, she did have a heart of gold and was pleased to be of help. She had seen Sylvia going out and then saw her drag herself back. Rose thought that she did not look well and when she saw the children run along the inside windowsill, she knew the mother was not aware of what they were doing, so she investigated. It was fortunate for all that she did come to the rescue.

When the doctor arrived, Nell explained her concern and they sent for a pediatric flying squad. The baby was transferred to Rotten Row's Special Care Baby Unit (SCBU) for observation.

Sylvia was upset at this, but understood that he was much too sleepy. Nell explained to her that a newborn baby should be wide-awake in the first hour after birth, but then he had had a rather fast descent into the world.

"I'll stay with Sylvia, Sister, till Craig gets home," said Rose.

"That is so good of you Rose. Well, I'll get on my way and Sister Bruce will see you in the morning Sylvia. I'll leave you the phone number for the SCBU."

"Craig will visit there before he comes home," said Sylvia.

Nell buttoned her double breasted coat, slipped the green belt through the bakelite buckle and pulled to tighten it, lifted her case and was on her way home.

Sister Bruce gave Nell an update on the Reid Family. Sylvia's young sister came through from Edinburgh to stay with her and Craig got home for two days compassionate leave before he had to go back to finish the course. The baby did not have a tentorial tear, as Nell had feared, but he did have meningitis, which was diagnosed quickly and treated. He was back home within three weeks.

Nell met Rose McPherson a few months later in Argyll Street as she was coming home from her weekly visit to the office in Ingram St.

"Hello Sister, how are you?"

"Oh hello Mrs. McPherson."

"Oh, just call me Rose. I'm out looking for a Christening gift for wee Craig Reid; they called him after his Daddy."

"That's nice; I was pleased that he did so well in hospital."

"Yes he is growing like a weed. I baby-sit for them and I am to be Craig's Godmother. The other children call me Aunty Rose." A big smile swept across Rose's face, she was brimming with pride.

"That's lovely, Rose you really saved the day, that day. It was so kind of you to step into the breech and look after everyone."

"Ocht Sister it was nothing. I was pleased to be of use for a change. My family have left home and my husband is at work all day, so I find time heavy on my hands."

"Have a nice Christening day Rose and give Sylvia my good wishes."

"Cheerio Sister, I'll do that for sure."

Nell walked on towards the bus stop. She was thinking of how people do need people; Nosey Rosey needed to feel needed and now that she did, she had changed to 'Aunty Rose'. It was a good thing, though, that Rosey was Nosey the day that Craig Reid was born.

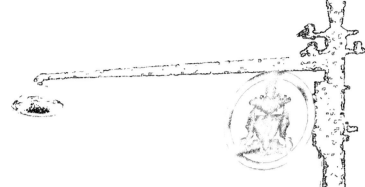

Chapter 18
Hazel Brown – Follow Up

Nell bumped into Hazel Brown as she was walking along Ingram Street in Glasgow, on her way back from her weekly visit to the Midwives Central Office. Hazel had just visited baby William in Rotten Row Hospital and Nell was on her way to the office.

"Have you time for a cuppa Hazel?" Nell asked. "Let me treat you for a change…I have not seen you for a couple of weeks now…"

"Well Ah have about half an hour before Ah need to head for the bus," Hazel said glancing at her wristwatch. "Well, OK then…that would be nice Sister. A cup o' char and a blether would be good… Ah was just going to get a snack before Ah head back home. Angie is watching the kids for me as Ah wanted to see the doctor this morning about wee William."

"So how is William doing?"

"Well he had a wee bit of a set back there, as he became quite anemic and they thought that he had internal bleeding. They think that he may have had that special bleeding that newborn babies get. Ah cannae mind what they cry it. They gave him more vitamin K and his blood count has been the same for the last two days. They had to give him some blood…that scared me…seein' the blood runnin' in tae him."

"How are his legs?" Nell inquired.

"Well he has them splinted now and I was hoping to take him home till the bleedin' happened."

"You are looking great Hazel…How is the rest of the family?"

"Oh they are all fine. I have been looking at a nursery school for Isabel to go to before she starts school. The head mistress in the school where I used to work came to see me and she has a friend who runs a nursery school. It is near to Bernie's work so he could take her in the morning and bring her home at lunch time three days a week. It will be good for Isabel. Hugh is fine. He just loves trains and fire engines, and would you believe it, Jess has started to walk now…and she is in at everything and keeps steeling Hugh's trains, the wee rascal!"

Hazel was full of her children's achievements and her face enlivened as she spoke about them. Nell was so pleased to see Hazel so talkative. Hazel was pleased to see Nell, as she always felt that she could talk freely with her. Nell was never judgmental.

They walked into the tearoom, slipped their coats off and made themselves comfortable at a small corner table. An order of two Russian teas and two rounds of egg and cress sandwiches were given. Nell had not had any lunch either so they were both rather peckish. Soon they were tucking into their snack and chatting freely.

"Hazel did you ever manage to find your father's family?"

"Did Ah ever Sister!…Wait till Ah tell you what happened…well ma Granny Blair told me where ma father's family used to live and Ah was able to trace them very quickly through an old neighbour!"

"That was amazing Hazel…go on I'm dying to hear how you got on."

"Well…this old neighbour, Sally, gave me the low-down on ma father. It turned out that ma father was a traveling salesman for a beer company and went all over Scotland. Unfortunately one of the hazards of the job was all the social drinking he was doing and he ended up with a drinking problem. He was in and out of jobs and was a bit of a vagabond. He never married till about three yeas ago when a widow woman with three teenage boys got her clutches intae him and he moved to her house in Mosspark…. You know right near Bellahouston Park."

"Yes it's very nice there," said Nell.

"But first Sister, Ah met Ma Granny MacLure. Old Sally invited me and ma Granny MacLure, one afternoon, tae her house."

"That was nice of her to do that for you Hazel."

"It was…it was really emotional though," said Hazel thoughtfully and tears welled in her eyes. "…but it was good and the next week we met there again with my Granny Blair and the kids…they all got on well because they knew each other from the old days before the MacLures moved away."

"There would've been a lot of blethering going on, eh?'"

"Oh sister it did ma heart good to see them with Beth, wee Hugh and Isobel…and the kids were like wee angels…you would have thought that butter wouldnae have melted in their mouths!"

"Funny how kids know when it's really important to be on good behaviour…isn't it?"

"It is that…and Ah found out that ma Granny MacLure lived in old Pollok with her son Brian and his wife Lynda. And wait till you hear this Sister…the truly amazing part is Sister," said Hazel quite excited "…Brian had dislocated hips and talipes when he was a baby and a small spina-bifida!"

"That is amazing Hazel…and how is he today?" asked Nell.

"Oh he is good…he walks with a cane and has a bad limp and a built up boot, but he is such a nice man and quite a character. When Bernie and I met him he had us in stitches laughing…and he and his wife want to keep in touch with us. So does old Granny MacLure…she is a dear, an' the ole' soul burst intae tears when I told her about William."

"That was great Hazel…look at the family you have now…and what about your father?" said Nell eagerly.

"Well sister…Ah did arrange tae meet him but it didnae go well at awe. Ah think he thought that Ah wanted money or something…but Ah got it off my chest and Ah told him a few home truths…and it won't bother me if Ah never see him again…but Ah left it that he would have tae make the next move. It was all worth it and I have the nice contact with Brian and Lynda and Granny MacLure. For years Ah thought that Ah was the reason that ma father didn't stay around."

"You must feel really great havin' done that…it must be so liberating."

"Sister…Ah tell ye…Ah havnae had that much satisfaction since a learned tae go a bike!" and she laughed out loud.

Hazel then turned her thoughts back to Baby William. "What dae ye call that—special baby bleedin', Sister? Angie will want to know when Ah get back…you know how she was a baby nurse…she has been a brick…and has more to do with the kids now…and they are gettin' used to seein' her."

"It is called haemolytic disease of the new born, and Angie will know it. It is caused by the baby not producing enough vitamin K. They can't produce vitamin K till the milk reaches the bowel…and babies who are sick often have intravenous drips…and are not fed milk for other reasons…" explained Nell.

"Oh ah see…thanks Sister."

"Here I'll write it on this envelope for you Hazel. It will be one less thing for you to remember."

"Great…thanks Sister…. Ah feel that ma brain is in overdrive!!!!"

"Well you are coping with a lot just now…How are you sleeping?"

"Oh better now than at the beginning…" Hazel replied "…. Ah phone the hospital last thing at night…you know that Angie and Joe got the phone put in the house for us…and Ah know all the nurses now…so Ah know that wee William is in good hands."

"It makes a difference to have a phone in the house," Nell agreed.

"Well if Bernie is working late, Ah don't feel so isolated…It's funny. Ah don't know how Ah managed without it!"

The two women finished their tea. Nell buttoned her coat, slipped the green belt through the green bakelite buckle, tugged to tighten it, and lifted her case ready to walk with Hazel toward the bus stop.

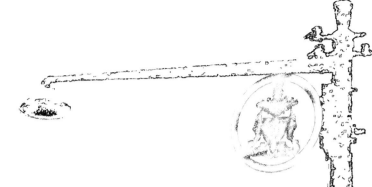

Chapter 19
Bridget Kelly's First Communion

Ever since the Reformation in 1560 there has been Catholic/Protestant rivalry in Glasgow. 'Rangers' in blue strips is the Protestant football team and 'Celtic' in Green strips is the catholic team. On Nell's first day at school when she was five, she came up against this rivalry. She was called a 'proddy dog.' Someone's big sister just told her to shout back 'kaflick cats'. She did not know what it meant, but did it anyway and it seemed to have the desired effect. Despite this rivalry, at grass roots if there was a human need everybody helped no matter what their religion. The Christian/ Jewish values ruled.

Nell was heading down the stairs of a tenement building in Gorbals. She glanced at her watch; nearly five o'clock. She better get a move on as it was almost closing time for the shops and she needed to buy some groceries.

As she got to the ground floor she could hear sobbing, "Oh my, someone is breaking their heart," thought Nell. On the ground floor there was the back close which led to the backcourt and back garden. The sobbing was louder there. Nell pushed open the back door. There, on a little wall, was a tiny human frame huddled down and crying hard. Nell recognized the beautiful mop of red curly hair. It was wee Bridget Kelly.

"Bridget, is that you? It's Sister Dickson, what has happened to you? Did you fall?"

"No Sister, I'm OK, really. It is jist that…" the tears blinded Bridget as her sobbing heaves started again. Nell bent over Bridget and put her hands on her shoulders.

"Come on Bridget, come with me," and Nell gave Bridget a large white laundered handkerchief. "Dry your eyes, hen, and tell me what's got you so upset." Nell sat down on the wall with her arm around Bridget.

"Well sister, the girls at school said that I would be the scabbiest girl in the first Communion procession because I have to wear my big cousin's dress; the one she had two years ago. My mammy can't afford to buy a new one and we don't know anyone who is going to Spain. Three girls in my class got absolutely beautiful dresses from Spain and they are all frills from head to toe."

"Bridget, I'm sure your cousin's dress can be fixed. I know a lady in the Baptist Church who could help. Is your Mammy in? Let's go and see her. It will be alright, you'll see."

"OK Sister, if you think it will be alright. I'll run and tell ma mammy you will be up to see her soon," and the mop of red hair bounced as a happier Bridget ran off.

Nell made a quick visit to Jeannie Ward who played the organ at the Baptist church. Nell had delivered Jeannie's sister last summer.

"Jeannie can you help a tragic situation?"

"Come on in Sister, the kettle is on the boil," Jennifer replied, as she invited Nell in.

Over a cup of tea they sorted out the problem of Bridget's dress. Nell would bring the existing dress to Jeannie and they would see what could be done. Jeannie had lots of wedding dress materials and plenty lace. Nell was very hopeful about the dress as she climbed the stairs to Mrs. Kelly's house, as she was thinking, how cruel kids can be to each other.

Mrs. Kelly was so pleased for the help.

"Oh Sister! Thank you so much. I jist don't have the extra cash at the moment. I'll be taking a few more closes to wash next month, so that will help. Since Tom died it's been tough. They promised compensation, but nothing so far."

Tom Kelly was killed in an accident at work. He was a plumber in a power station. Mrs. Kelly (Bridie) was left with three children; Bridget was the eldest.

"I think that Jeannie will do a good job of the dress," Nell reassured Bridie Kelly.

"Oh I'm sure she will. I saw a wedding dress that she made and it was just lovely," said Bridie.

The 'bush telegraph' was at work and soon Jeannie Ward was swamped with lovely pieces of white satin and brocade and lots of pieces of white lace.

"Sister you wouldn't believe it, come in and see for yourself!" Jeannie when she met Nell later that week.

"That is wonderful, Jeannie I'm so pleased; people are so kind," replied Nell as a tear came to her eye at the thought.

"They sure want wee Bridget to be the nicest. The wee soul lost her daddy last year," said Jeannie.

Work had begun on the dress and Nell popped in to see Jeannie most mornings. Jeannie was so excited, as she was trusted to do the work.

One morning, Nell left the bakery with six treacle crumpets in a paper bag. She headed for Jeannie Ward's place. The smell of the crumpets was filling the air as Jeannie opened the door. "Oh Sister, the tea's just masked come in…what have you got there?" Jennie gestured at the baker's bag of goodies.

"Just a wee 'chittering bite' on a cold morning," Nell laughed.

"Come in, come away in and we will get our jaws wrapped round these crumpets, I'll get the butter and Jam," laughed Jeannie.

After the tea Jeannie, held up the dress for all to see. There were gasps of surprise from thee five ladies gathered there. The dress was absolutely lovely!

"A sheer transformation, Jeannie." Nell said.

The other ladies showered Jeannie with praise. Nell looked around the group. She knew most of them. She was pleased to see there were two ladies from the 'Catholic Mother's Union' as well as the rest from the Baptist Church and the Parish Church. 'Community spirit,' Nell thought, as she brushed the tears from her eyes.

Nell collected Bridie Kelly and Bridget Kelly later that day and they headed for Jeannie Ward's place to have a wee peak at the dress. Bridget looked a treat in the dress and she loved it.

"Those lasses in my class can't call this scabby, can they Mammy?" Bridget beamed.

"No hen, they canny do that. It is a beautiful dress and you look like a princess in it." Bridie answered proudly as she hugged her daughter. It was a happy scene.

"Thanks Jeannie, you have a special gift," said Bridie,

"Thank you very much, Mrs. Ward," said Bridget and she gave Jeannie a kiss on the cheek.

"That's alright hen, I was pleased to help. You just have a lovely day!" replied Jeannie, with a tear in her eye.

Everyone clapped and sang "for she's a jolly good fellow" as they circled Jeannie. Jeannie beamed a big smile. She was pleased it had all worked out so well.

Nell left the happy scene. She walked along the road and heard someone call her name. She turned round and saw Manny Needleman waving to her. This was the father of one of her patients whom she delivered a few months ago. He ran a successful tailoring business. He often offered Nell a stack of boy's school trousers that needed to be sewn up. He knew she would know the families in need.

"Hello Manny, how are you?" greeted Nell, "and how is that grandson, Eric?"

"I'm fine Sister, and the baby is doing well. How did the communion dress work out?" asked Manny.

"Oh it's lovely, but how did you know?" Nell inquired, amazed, as always at the efficiency of the grapevine.

" Two of my best seamstresses know Jeannie Ward." Manny explained. "Tell me, Nell, has the wee lassie got a cloak for the day?"

"No I don't think she has" relied Nell.

"Well, come round to the factory tomorrow. I think I may have a nice piece of satin lining in a sapphire blue colour that may do the trick. That's the wee lassie with the red hair, am I right?" Manny asked.

"Yes it is. Bridget is her name," said Nell.

"Aye I remember her father. He helped me out when I had a flood in the factory last year. He was a good wee man and I would like to see his wee lassie look the best," smiled Manny.

"Thanks Manny! You are a real gent." Nell said, as she picked up her case, tightened the belt of her green coat and was on her way.

Nell remembered when she first met Manny. It was the birth of his grandson Eric. Nell gave Manny the baby to hold just after he was born. Although he had had twelve children of his own, he has never held a newborn. Manny was thrilled with baby Eric.

A week later there was a beautiful hooded cloak for Bridget Kelly. Her red hair framed her face and her red curls, which, in turn, was framed by the blue satin hood of her new cloak. The local hairdresser, Sylvia, offered to fix the hood onto Bridget's hair with glittery clasps.

The day arrived and the community turned out to see all the children filing into the chapel. Bridget was stunning and the sapphire cloak shimmered in the morning sun. She was a star and certainly far from shabby or scabby. Bridget smiled brightly on her First Communion Day, with the love and concern her community had showered upon her, and her mammy was as proud of her as her daddy would have been.

There was hardly a dry eye amongst those who were watching the procession. Nell saw Manny walk past and she gave him a wave. He returned a 'thumbs up' to Nell and his big beaming smile said "we did it!"

Nell thought, 'Thanks to Zeida Needleman. You helped make Bridget's day.'

Nell made her way to the bus stop. She fastened her coat, put the green belt through the green buckle and pulled to tighten it, dusted off her case and was on her way to her next visit.

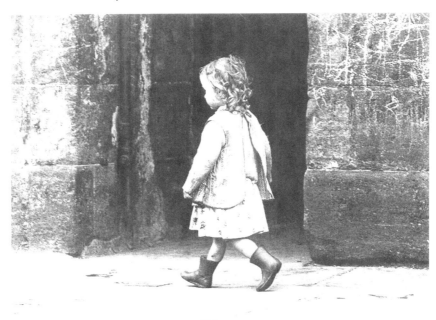

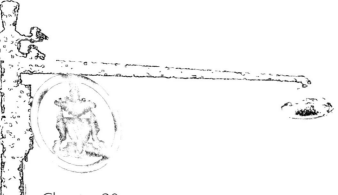

Chapter 20
George's Patsy

A shaft of light pierced the pitch dark of the bedroom through a chink in the heavily lined velvet curtains. It fell on George's sleeping eyes. He stirred. He sank back into the pillow, aware now that she was in a quiet slumber and he relaxed. George was truly thankful her bouts of vomiting had finally ceased. It was probably that prawn cocktail that they had last night at the staff party. His eyes feasted on her silhouette. She was so fragile looking, like porcelain doll with alabaster paleness with peach tinges, delicately featured, beautifully crafted, graceful in form, a tangible work of art.

His heart throbbed into his throat with sheer love for Patsy and tears of emotion welled up in his eyes. He gently stroked the silky tresses of her long dark hair that were strewn over the pillows and his eyes followed the curve of her slender back. He had never known such deep feelings as this before; it seemed to encompass all the love he had ever known multiplied ten thousand times. The love that he once had for his wife, Sue, and the fatherly love he had for Christine and Fiona, plus all the fervent love affairs over the years, seemed to pale in significance when he thought of his feelings for Patsy.

She besotted him; she was ever present in his consciousness. He rarely stayed late at school now. He was always eager to get home to her and often came bearing some tasty treat, some pretty flowers or some wee quirky gift.

He gulped and swallowed hard, wiped the sleep and tears away with the backs of both hands in a cat-like motion and quietly rose out of bed. He donned a paisley patterned silk robe, a present from Patsy, slipped his feet into leather mules, also a present from Patsy, and tip toed towards the bedroom door. He would let her sleep undisturbed and with a last longing look towards his sleeping beauty, he closed the door behind him.

George awaited the kettle boiling. He had kept the whistling part off the spout so as not to waken Patsy with Billy's whistle. He smiled as he could hear Patsy say, "There's whistling Billy," when the kettle boiled. He just loved all her little sayings and habits.

She loved to sit crossed legged on the sofa with her hands wrapped round a steaming mug of tea and bathe her face in the rising vapours. That was it! She made the everyday things special and almost magical. He wanted to be with her every minute of the day just watching her. Her mannerisms made his heart sing. They had not had much time together lately, as the run up to Christmas at their respective schools was chaotic, to say the least. Now they had the Christmas holidays to get things back on track and he looked forward to doing just that. He loved living with Patsy and the last three months since Sue ordered him out had been good.

Sue had made it so easy for him that he could not believe his luck. Out of his wife's house into his lover's house in one swift move! No hassles. The notion of being a kept man briefly entered his thoughts but was dismissed immediately. After all, he did pay his way. He paid half of Patsy's mortgage payment and housekeeping bills and they were planning to buy a house together when his divorce from Sue was final. Patsy would not believe that George had no stake in Sue's Pollokshield home. He told her repeatedly that the house was willed to Sue by her grandmother and was clearly stated that George would never own it or part of it. Patsy said that she had a friend who was a lawyer and she would get him to look into George's rights.

George had never had to pay a mortgage payment when he was with Sue, which was one reason he could afford to run about in the latest model of Austin Princess and have a membership to Hagg's Castle Golf Club. There would be no new car next year and his golf membership may have to lapse, but then Patsy, his "passionate pie," was his handicap now and he much preferred it that way. He warmed all over at the thought of Patsy and her fervent passion and it was a bonus to him, not a handicap at all!

He rinsed the teapot with boiling water then made the tea while he put a couple of slices of plain bread under the grill to toast. He collected the mail and the morning paper from behind the door and threw them on the table in time to rescue the toast—which was a near thing! He didn't want to waken Patsy with the smell of burned toast. He glanced at the headlines in the Glasgow Herald…the police getting a wage hike. Lucky buggers, he thought, and then went straight for the crossword section of the paper. This was the life! It was a ritual now; tea, buttered toast with a wee smear of thick cut marmalade and the morning crossword.

When he lived with Sue, there was no time for such luxuries. There was always such chatter at the breakfast table and the girls were the center of all the attention, what they were doing that day after school etc. Yes he did miss them in some ways, but a wry smile crossed his face when he thought of his life with Patsy. Life was easy and good. They planned to travel this summer to Rome, Paris and Athens. Yes! They were free to wonder round the wonders of Europe. He beamed broadly as the holiday spirit encompassed him.

George leaned back on the legs of the kitchen chair and swayed to and fro, the pencil resting lightly on his right ear while he munched the black crust of the toast. A six-letter word meaning "kept man or professional dancing partner"…he already had the last three letters "o-l-o"…He leaned forward and entered "g-i-g" in the squares. He stared at the word. A kept man…a gigolo…is that what he had become? This was Patsy's flat but he did pay his share and his dancing could certainly not be called professional! He smiled at the mental picture of his dancing and the "gigolo" thought dimmed, but that was twice in one morning the "kept man concept" had entered his consciousness. He moved on to the next clue. "Excellently well dressed"…five letters, beginning with "d" and ending with "y". Of course! And he penciled in the letters "and", making "dandy". He stared at the word and immediately he could hear his mother's voice in one of her many tirades, "…you strut about like Burlington Bertie with nothing to back it up either!…Just a dandy you are!…Get some sense George and appreciate Sue and your two great girls before it is too late…you will rue the day if you don't…!"

George threw the paper aside. He usually enjoyed the crossword, but not today. A feeling of restlessness swept over him. Perhaps he needed to make a move and buy a different place with Patsy or at least legally share this one. He wished that Patsy would not go on about him being entitled to part of Sue's house in Pollokshields. She was hinting at them buying a new house in Bearsden. He would have to tell her once and for all that he will have to save for a down payment on another house and there will be no payment to him from Sue.

He would have to phone Sue today, as he had promised to take the girls to the circus at Kelvin Hall and then on to the fun fair afterwards. This was one thing that he had always done with them, although Christine could hardly bear to speak to him since that night in the Samaritan Hospital when Sue nearly died from an ectopic pregnancy. But Fiona was still quite chatty to him on the phone. Patsy would come too and they would have a family outing and, as it was totally in public, Christine could not be too rude to Patsy, he hoped. Children brought their own set of problems, that was for sure…perhaps the week between Christmas and the New Year would be best for the circus outing. He would go over on Christmas Eve day to take the gifts and see his mother and sister at the same time.

It was a peculiar arrangement with his mother and sister living with his ex-wife and daughters. It was a totally strange estrangement! They were all strong women he mused, except for his sister who was mentally handicapped. Patsy needed him more. He always thought of her as delicate and requiring protection and he liked the feeling that gave him as her protector. Yes, he was happy with his lot. He proceeded to feed Patsy's two Siamese cats. They were less trouble than children were, he mused, and so independent! The cats watched him from afar and took their time to sidle over to their respected dishes to eat. They too had sized up George Taylor.

He walked through to the front of the house and looked out of the lounge bay window upon the scene below. Overnight the hard frost had dressed the place a coat of white; the leafless tree skeletons glimmered pink where the low morning sun caught them. The hustle and bustle of a Glasgow morning was well under way, with pedestrians dodging each other in the busyness of Byres Road, which George could just see at the end of the street, amongst white vapour clouds issuing forth into the frosty air with each breath they took. Scarves abounded in diverse colours. Broad stripes adorned men's necks, the checkered head-square variety securely tied under the women's chins and hands hidden in gloves.

A tram car rattling down Byres Road jostled its passengers to and fro as it gathered speed and there seemed to be a swell of people in the street all of a sudden, probably from the underground station, all bustling about rushing to work, no doubt. Four young ladies with black clad legs were hurrying towards the Western Infirmary. What nursing feats lay before them today, George wondered? Perhaps they will save the life of a child, be kind to a lonely man, or aid in the latest ground breaking surgery.

The clinking of milk bottles brought George back from his day dreaming. There below him was a milk float with a couple of boys hanging onto its back as it shuddered over the cobble stones of the street on its way back to the Scottish Farmer's depot. George smiled at the boys as they swung about chattering to each other. He could even make out the grins on their faces. Long may they be as carefree as they are at this moment, but one never knew the stories behind the faces.

George's heart missed a beat as one of the milk boys almost fell off the float. Boys will be boys, he thought as he watched them…and wondered if the baby that Sue lost would have been a boy…a lost boy. He would have liked a son…what would he have become? The Milk float with its interesting cargo trundled round onto Byres Road and disappeared from George's sight, and the distinctive rattle of the milk bottles against the crates faded from his earshot. George turned with his thoughts inward to the room.

It was a large room, sparsely furnished. There in the corner was Patsy's easel with a canvas in readiness for a potentially wonderful work of art. The large long wall was bare of furniture. That was it! He would buy a piece of furniture for this room. Something modern would be nice. If Patsy felt up to it they could have a look today. He felt instantly more relieved now, with this plan of action. That's what they needed, things that were theirs, things that they purchased together, things that had their stamp. After all they were a couple, an item and a family. He felt elated as he strode purposely toward the bathroom for his morning ablutions. He finished by splashing an ample amount of Yardley after-shave lotion on his jaw-line. He hissed through his teeth as the lotion stung a nick on his chin…he glanced in the mirror to inspect the tiny wound and there he saw a sleepy Patsy behind him. He swung round and encased her in his arms.

"You smell divinely devilish George, mmm…" She snuggled into him.

"You look wicked angel girl…"

They both laughed as they hugged tightly, each not wanting to release their hold, as it felt so comfortably comforting. Then George kissed the top of Patsy's head and said, "I have a plan for today and I hope you will like it."

"Oh can it be a surprise!…Like a mystery tour…please, please, Georgie," Sue pleaded in a childish voice.

"You're definitely on…I shall be your tour guide for today…shall I run you a bath, Madam?" said George in a butler's bow.

"Oh do I stink that bad?"

"Not at all, my darling," fibbed George, as there was a slight stale lingering odour of vomit from her hair. "I was only trying to be of service Madam," continued George in his butler's mode.

"Well a bath would be lovely…I do feel a bit sticky and I need to brush my teeth…thank goodness I feel better now. I will never eat prawns again as long as I live."

George put the plug in the bath, threw a bath cube in and soon the hot water was splattering from the wide brass spout. He also switched on the wall heater.

"Come and I'll make you some fresh tea and toast." They both approached the kitchen.

"I'll have breakfast after my bath I think. Thanks…I'll just have some Lucosade and a cracker just now, to keep my tummy settled." Patsy poured a shot glass of the amber tonic and took a cracker from the tartan biscuit tin. Cracker between her teeth and glass in hand, she headed for the now steamy bathroom, where the cats were already in their positions. One was nestling on a thick folded bath towel that lay at the bottom end of the bath and the other was erect in a guard-like position atop of the white wicker bathroom chair. All was well; the cats were in control.

Patsy stepped, toe–first, into the steaming rose-perfumed water and gradually lowered body into the bath. She lay there with the cats watching her every move. Patsy admired her cats. They appear so mystical in their stillness, she thought, as if they know a secret, as if they can see into the future. That vomiting was something else! She had never known anything like that before. She couldn't be pregnant…no…she had been told that she would never be able to have children. That was one reason her first husband left her…she didn't tell George that as it wouldn't matter to him anyway. He was a father already and he always wore a sheath.

Suddenly she sat bolt upright in the bath…both cats startled and rose to all fours. Oh no, that student art teacher Adam! That impromptu lustful sex…the heat of the moment fling, when she was studying his portfolio! That happened just before George arrived to stay, the night Sue told him to leave. No! No! No!…It was the prawns…she did not even like the taste of them…She could not be pregnant and that was that…Perish that thought.

Soon they were in the thick of the traffic heading for Glasgow City centre. George loved to drive his silver Austin Princess and Patsy felt like a Lady in the front passenger seat. She had on a red fitted coat with black fur round the collar, cuffs and hem with matching accessories; a black fur hat with a red trim, black leather gloves with red stitching, and a black leather handbag. Patsy's boots were her newest acquisition. They were knee length, high-heeled boots in soft black leather. All in all she made a fashion statement, which George adored. George wore his heavy grey Crombie coat and grey leather driving gloves. A blue checked scarf peeked out under the coat collar and accented the muted blues in his soft hat. He liked wearing a hat, as it gave him extra height and hid his receding hairline. One could say they were well clad!

"Open your eyes now Patsy…surprise!" said George guiding her into a furniture shop. "What do you like the best…this…this…or this…for the lounge?" George swept his hand as he spoke showcasing some modern expensive teak furniture.

"Oh George what a surprise!…This stuff is just beautiful…I love the richness and depth in the teak…Oh yes, I just adore this unit and I think it will sit well on the bare wall of our lounge."

George was so pleased that she said "our lounge" that he almost purred aloud. Patsy decided on a sideboard unit and a matching coffee table. The coffee table was six feet long and had shelves suitable for Patsy's large Illustrated Art Books. George settled the bill and arranged for the delivery of the furniture the following Monday. They left the car and walked along toward Argyle Street. Patsy snuggled into George, her right arm through his left and her left hand hanging on too. The next surprise was that George swung her into a Travel Bureau.

"Patsy we are going to pick up some brochures to look through over the holidays and we are going to have a European holiday of a lifetime this summer."

"George I do love you and I have always wanted to see Rome and Athens."

"Well we are free agents, Patsy. All you have to do is get your mother to look after the cats and we will have two months in Europe…wherever you wish."

"I almost feel giddy with happiness," said Patsy, euphorically. "I feel as if I am floating on air."

George smiled widely. This was going well. He felt better now and his morning feeling of inadequacy had left him. Patsy was enjoying herself too. George was pleased. They left the Travel Bureau and continued arm in arm. He felt that he was in control and calling the shots and that made him feel manly.

"Now for your real Christmas present…a new dress…let's hit some dress shops."

"George you are amazing. How did you know that I was thinking of a new dress for Christmas?" smiled Patsy.

George used to hate this type of shopping in the ladies' dress stores, with the eager sales assistants who would say anything to get a sale.

"Doesn't madam look gorgeous in that," or "That's just you to a tee," or "Look at this young lady Maud," (calling on a colleague)…"Have you ever seen anything as perfect?…It brings out the colour in your eyes dearie." When they got really desperate, out would come, "Well you'll never get anything as good as that for the price…I mean to say it really is the store bargain and the only one left in your size."

Things were different shopping with Patsy. She was so keen to try different things. She loved gay colours and patterns and George loved to see her emerge from the dressing rooms in the various modes, she was a treat to behold and her trim figure was easy to fit. In one of the big department stores, she was asking George his opinion. He did not like the black dress, as it seemed to make her look pale…drew the colour from her face.

She turned to him. "How do I look?" When Patsy gave a pirouette she stumbled, and George rushed to catch her before she fell to the floor. Two assistants rushed with a chair and a cup of water. An ashen-faced Patsy was helped into a dressing room that had a window opening to the outside.

"Give her some fresh air," said the manageress who was now taking control of the situation, "Call for the First Aid attendant Louise," she said to the sales assistant. "Now dear, try to put your head between your legs," she said to Patsy as she yanked Patsy's head down to her knees.

"I think I am OK now, we should have stopped for some lunch…we have been shopping for hours," said Patsy.

The manageress left Patsy with Louise and the First Aid attendant. She asked George if he had a car. "Well, I think you should bring the car to the back door and we will take her down there, on the wheel chair, to meet you."

"It will take me about twenty minutes to get there and bring the car back. You won't leave her on her own?" George queried.

"Don't worry about a thing, I realize your concern Sir. So…congratulations are in order…When is the baby due?" smiled the manageress with a wink and nod of her head.

"Oh she's not pregnant…it was the prawns that she ate last night."

"Oh well she will be fine soon," said the manageress as she shooed George out of the department toward the lift. She rolled her eyes upward when George was out of sight, "Prawns my Aunty Fanny…she's preggers all right, it is as plain as the nose on his face…and them not married either…Oh well that's life!" She muttered under her breath as she made her way back to see how Patsy and her department were doing.

The furniture arrived and Christmas was a wonderful celebration. They took the girls to the Kelvin Hall Circus and Christine was predictably rude to Patsy, while Fiona was charming. Patsy's family visited and they liked the teak furniture, but the drowsiness and sickness persisted. The New Year dawned with a round of parties and visiting friends, and still the sickness persisted. Then there was a visit to the doctor, medication, and another visit to the doctor. A baby expected at the end of July!

George was astounded! How could this have happened? He had taken special precautions. He would stand by her of course, but it was rotten timing! If only they had waited. If only he was free to marry her. If only he had some control over this situation. What a fool he had been…prawns indeed! He felt his face go crimson when he thought back to his day shopping with Patsy! Those women must have known. Women know these things. Patsy didn't; or was that denial. George thought hard. No…she was not involved with anyone else…there was no time…he was sure of that. This was his baby and he would face up to his responsibilities. He smiled at the thought of Patsy being a mother…and perhaps he would get his son? But what of their holiday plans?

A couple of mundane months passed. He stared at the floor, head in hands, elbows on knees and gut in spasm. It was a surreal moment. He was worried about Patsy. Her sickness had worsened and he had insisted on phoning an ambulance and here they were in Glasgow Royal Maternity Hospital, (Rotten Row). Patsy was to be admitted. He breathed deeply as he thought of her pale thin, fragile face, and he prayed for help. One thing they did say that the foetal heart was strong, but Patsy would need replacement fluids and electrolytes. He sat up rubbing his forehead and Patsy's mother appeared in the distant corridor. This was a vision that George could do without at this moment!

Esmie and her husband, Art, approached. She was the same cut as

Patsy, but ruled with a rod of iron. George could see that she was fuming, even from a distance. Art walked behind her at a safe pace; he was henpecked in the extreme although he was a big man. He followed like the calm after the storm.

"I just heard about this pregnancy last week…what were you thinking and you a married man with children. Where is the sense in all this?…Assistant headmaster into the bargain! Wait till this gets round the school…some example you are for your own children and your pupils…acting like a pair of love sick teenagers…and I warned her that if she played with fire she would get burned…see my words have come true. Just you wait till I see her I will give her a piece of my mind…why has she done this to me? What a mother has to put up with…what did I do to deserve this?" Esmie suddenly stopped the tantrum to dab her nose and eyes with a purple spotted handkerchief and take some deep breaths in.

"Now Esmie, it's not all that bad. I think that you're making a mountain out of a mole hill," offered Art.

"A mountain out of a mole hill indeed! Your head's in the clouds, Art and always has been…just the same as Patsy's."

George had about all he could take of this charade and he rose to his feet. "Esmie please sit down here," he pointed to the bench where he had been sitting. "Art please have a seat," again George gestured toward the bench. "I have something very important to tell you both…"

The solemn look on George's face quelled Esmie's high horse and Art tentatively put his arm round her as they sat down together looking up into George's eyes.

George cleared his throat. "I love Patsy very much." He paused. "We did not plan this pregnancy and I am really worried about her condition. Her vomiting has been too severe and the doctor called it Hyperemesis Gravidarum…It means too much vomiting in pregnancy. They have to keep her in and give her intravenous fluids and electrolytes. They have to stop the vomiting. I wish I could make it all better for her but I feel so helpless. I can only love her and give her all my support." He looked at them with tears in his eyes. The two concerned faces stared back with ever widening eyes.

"Oh my wee lassie," said Esmie, "I didn't know she was in any danger…and the baby?"

"Strong heartbeat," said George trying to smile.

"OK then," said Art, "we are with you George, and we will all get through this…Now Esmie, it will be easier for Patsy if she sees us all friends." He patted George on the back.

Esmie offered a hand to George. "Truce?"

"Truce it is Esmie, and thanks," George took Esmie's hands and gave her a wee peck on the cheek. She blushed with pleasure.

"I won't let your lassie down, we will be married the day my divorce comes through."

Esmie opened her mouth to say something, but Art interrupted her thought with, "Enough said Esmie…When can we see Patsy, George?"

"They are just waiting for some blood test results and a drip to be put into her arm. They could not find a decent vein, so the anesthetist is going to do it, then they are taking her to Ward 5. I think it is just along that corridor to the left on the ground floor."

George pointed along the long clinically clean corridor. The smell of pine disinfectant was getting to him and he felt distinctively nauseated! He walked slowly and determinedly with Esmie and Art in tow, toward the front door of the hospital for some fresh air. The front hall porter opened the door for them when he saw George's ashen face.

"Over here sir, you can sit on the wall and get some fresh air."

Esmie and Art flanked George as he sat there. A somewhat solemn trio, George thought. Oh Patsy, please pull though, George prayed.

Patsy did pull through and the remainder of her pregnancy went well. She booked a home confinement and gave birth to a baby boy on midsummer's night. George was an integral part of the proceedings and fussed over Patsy and son like an old mother hen. Mother and baby were well and they called the baby Garry, although Patsy wanted to call him Puck. He was small, weighing in at five pounds eleven ounces. Garry was three days old when Nell called to do an afternoon visit. She had not seen George Taylor since the night he drove her home from booking Sue for a home confinement, about a year before.

Nell was taken aback when George opened the door to her ring.

"Come in Sister…They are both in the bedroom. My daughters are visiting their half brother for the first time." George had not recognized Nell in the darkened hallway. Nell walked into the large bedroom and there before her was Patsy lying in bed with the Moses' basket close to her and Christine and Fiona looking down at the baby.

"He's so wee," said Fiona. "Look at the size of his fingers."

"He's only half a brother," said Christine under her breath, "what do you expect Fiona?" she said in a normal voice. Christine turned round and saw Nell. "Hello Sister Dickson, I did not think that you came to this side of the river…nice to see you."

"Hello Christine and Fiona. So, you have a beautiful little brother here," said Nell quickly computing the situation.

"He's our half brother," said Christine on the defensive.

Nell quickly turned to Patsy. "I'm Sister Dickson. I'm here to see you, as Sister Black has been called to a confinement…How are you doing?"

"Fine I think, just a bit tired…. We have to feed him every three hours…but sometimes he isn't really interested…I hope he is gaining weight OK…Sister Black is going to weigh him tomorrow."

"Now girls, can you go into the other room till I am finished here? Then you can come back in," said Nell smiling at Christine and Fiona.

"OK," chorused the girls as they made for the door and their dad.

The whole story came flooding back to Nell. This must be Patsy the art teacher, the one that Sue Taylor had told her about. It was a small world and the odds of Nell paying a visit on Patsy were high. There was Patsy looking exhausted with this wee scrag of a baby. Nell looked at Garry Taylor who had no strong resemblance to mother or father. He was cute though, and would come on a treat. Most of the small babies did well with the proper care, attention and love. Nell was sure that this cherub would receive all of these.

Nell performed a postnatal check on Patsy and chatted to her as she did so. Patsy burst into tears and sobbed quietly.

Nell handed her some tissues. "Just let it all out Patsy, it's OK to cry." Nell sat beside Patsy and lifted baby Garry on her knee. He was a lightweight. She unwrapped him to check his temperature and cord stump. She applied purple methylated spirit to the cord stump, applied powder and changed the cord dressing, reapplying a length of crepe bandage as a binder round the baby to keep the dressing in place.

"Remember Patsy, if this gets wet, put on another, but not tightly…just like this," and she let Patsy feel the bandage. "The cord is drying nicely and I'm sure it will fall off in about another five days."

"I don't like to touch it Sister…" sniffed Patsy, "I'm afraid it hurts him…he always cries when I do it."

"You can't hurt him Patsy, as there are no nerves there, but they often cry as the sprit is cold on their skin."

"Is there anything in specific that is bothering you?" said Nell as she cleared away the sodden paper hankies.

"Oh it's just Christine. She does not like me and she always manages to upset me…it will pass. George gets angry with her and then there's a row…and she goes home in the huff," explained Patsy.

"That's Christine's problem and she will have to deal with it…don't you upset yourself…You have this little man to take care of now. How is the feeding going?" Nell inquired.

"Well…" said Patsy picking up a pad of paper to show Nell the feeding record, "I am offering him the breast every second feed but I also top him up after a breastfeed. He is a hungry wee soul when he starts, but soon falls asleep…I only hope he is getting enough, as I don't want him to go into hospital."

Nell looked at the feeding record. "I think he is getting enough. The three hourly feeds makes a difference when they are this small. He is due a feed now. How do you feel about Christine feeding him? Did you know she is going to be a nurse? I will stay and supervise her."

"OK Sister, if you will stay for the feed I could do with a sleep, I'm fair wabbitt." Patsy slid down in the bed and curled on her side. "Thanks Sister, hope to see you again."

Nell wheeled the Moses basket through the large hallway towards the lounge. She overheard George saying, "I don't want to hear you call your brother a bastard again Christine…that makes me very sad."

"I didn't call him that Dad. I only said that the dictionary definition for a baby born out of wedlock was "illegitimate" or "bastard". I did not call Garry that," said Christine, in her own defense.

Christine is pushing George's buttons, Nell thought.

"Hello there, here comes a baby," Nell called to warn them of her approach.

"Come in sister. I did not recognize you when I opened the door to you. I just really saw the green uniform…" George apologized.

"Oh don't worry about that…one Green Lady looks very much like the next," said Nell nonchalantly. "Patsy desperately needs to sleep and wondered if Christine would feed Garry for her." Nell lifted Garry and gave him to Christine.

Christine flushed, but took the baby and sat down. "I hope that he does not choke or anything. I have never fed a baby this young before…"

"Don't worry, I will stay with you and perhaps Fiona will hold him for a while after he has fed, to make sure he brings up all his wind…He's a precious wee mite, isn't he Christine?"

"I'll get the bottle ready," said George.

Christine gazed down at the tiny frame of her half brother as she fed him and thought, Garry Taylor you are my very own wee brother. I think I love you very much. Tears trickled down Christine's face but she kept her head bowed for the longest time.

"Thank you Sister…for everything…" said a tired looking George. "Perhaps we will see you again?"

"Perhaps," said Nell as she buttoned her green coat and slid the green belt through the green bakelite buckle, tugged to tighten it, lifted her case and was on her way. She never saw George Taylor or Patsy again.

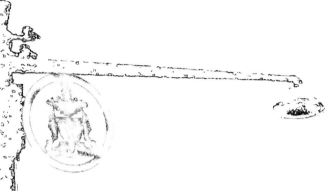

Epilogue

In the 1960s, I had three children of my own. One of my colleagues, a Green Lady, delivered my first baby in 1965 at home in Shawlands; a son who, unfortunately, died at the age of twenty-one. Four years later, after a brisk hemorrhage, I had a section in Rotten Row for placenta previa. Morag Anne has given me two beautiful grandchildren, Rebecca and Jamie. They live in Australia. In 1971, following an induction, I had a forceps delivery of Sheila who is now a midwife in Wales. Both daughters trained to be nurses.

Looking back over my life and work, I have been blessed to have had such a rewarding career. I loved my work as a Green Lady. It was a way of life, as the twenty four-hour call, five and a half days per week, meant that it was your life. Being so involved with the mothers from early pregnancy to the postnatal period, I learned so much from them.

— Helena Joyce

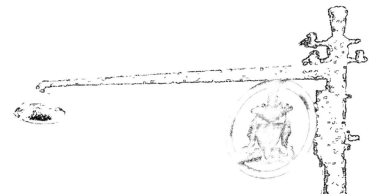

Glossary

Word or Expression	Meaning
a bit wabbit	a little tired
a wee doad	a little bit
act daft and get a free hurl	act crazy and get a free ride
aw the lolly	ah the money
awffy	awfully
baith	both
ball would have been on the slates	end of the game
blether	to chat incessantly
blethered	gabbed or talked on
boak	to be sick to one's stomach
broat	brought
bunnet	bonnet, cap or hat
cannae whack	can't beat that
caul	membrane over a newborn's head
close	the hallways and stairs of a tenement building
cor	car
crombie coat	heavy woolen coat
dae	do
dinna fash	don't fuss
dinna fash yersel	don't have to fuss
domiciliary	community or district
dreep	a drip

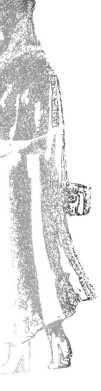

Word or Expression	Meaning
dreeped down off the midden	hang by the finger tips and jump off a wall
driech day	rotten weather
efter	after
erse frae	ass from
Faither	Father
fitba	football or soccer
flanny sheets	flannel sheets
frae	from
frilled pinny	frilly apron
gie, gied, gies	give, gave, give me
glaekit	a bit simple or stupid looking
glaur	glare at
Gorbals	District in Glasgow south side
gritty	stamina or strength
guff	muck
hame	home
heed	head
hert	heart
hing out the windae	hang out the window
hingin'	hanging
hingin'oot	hanging out
his wullie's awefie wee	his penis is awfully small
hoaspital	hospital
hoat	hot
Hogmanay	New Years Eve
hoose	house
Hungry Horaces	Hungry Horace was a comic character who could eat a lot
hurl	ride: 'act daft and get a free hurl'
jeely	jelly or jam
jeely piece	jam sandwich

Glossary

Word or Expression	Meaning
jist	just
knickers	underwear (panties)
lang	long
limpet	limp
loast	lost
loat	a lot
lolly	money or cash
lorry	truck
lying stotious	lying drunk
ma	my or mother
mair	more
ménage	payment scheme for goods
middin	bin or garbage can
minnit	minute
nae	no
nat	that
naw	no
nawallno, naw-al-no	no I will not; 'no I not'
noo	now
oan	own
oot	out
oxters	armpits
parkie	park keeper
peely wally	pale or washed out looking
play piece	snack for school recess
posseted milk	baby spit-up milk
purrich	porridge
ra	the
rounders	American Football
shoap	shop
sister dora caps	squareish starched nurses cap
sters	stairs

Word or Expression	Meaning
ta ta the noo	bye bye for now
tae swallae	to swallow
tatties	potatoes
the wrang wans	the wrong ones
totties	potatoes
treacle scones	scones made with molasses
wabbit	exhausted
waberian style	strict management style
wally	clay
wally dugs	clay dogs
watter	water
wauchle	waddle
wean	child
weans	childen
wee cherub	little children with angel like faces
wee poor waifs	poor scruffy children
wee yins	little ones
whit	what
wi	with
wid	would
wis	was
Wrigley's birthing forceps	small obstectricle forceps
yer	your
yersel	yourself
yi	you
yir	your

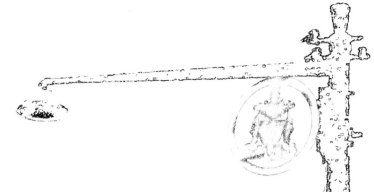

About The Author

Helena Joyce grew up in the North, then the South West of Glasgow. She completed a three year nursing program at the Southern General Hospital in Glasgow, followed by a 'first part' midwifery program at the Rankin Memorial in Greenock. She returned to the Southern General where she completed the 'second part' of her midwifery education, that had a strong district component in an area of Glasgow called Govan.

After a brief time working with 'Queens District Nursing in Glasgow', she gained employment as a 'Glasgow Corporation Domiciliary Midwife', lovingly referred to by the Glasgow people as 'green ladies' because of their green uniforms. In the 1970s, Helena completed a Midwifery Tutor's Diploma (MTD) and taught midwifery at Glasgow Southern College and the 'new' Rutherglen Maternity Hospital. This was the beginning of her career as a maternity care educator.

Helena immigrated to British Columbia, Canada in 1987, where she was well received into maternity nursing. Her experience and depth of knowledge were quickly recognized and she was asked to write seventeen educational modules for an 'Advanced Obstetrical Nursing Specialty' course for maternity nurses. This course was the nearest that BC had to a midwifery education program at that time. BC now has a recognized Midwifery program, established in 2002 at the University of British Columbia.

While living in the Fraser Valley in BC, Helena advanced her own education by completing a Bachelor of Science in Nursing and a Masters Degree in Education. Her involvement in education continued, as a lecturer in a general nursing program, teaching the maternity content. She retired to Vancouver Island in 2004 and moved to Ladysmith BC, where she a co-founded the Ladysmith Writers' Circle. However, she was soon enticed back to work by the lack of nursing lecturers at Malaspina University College, where she taught maternity nursing until the time of her death in December 2008.

The Green Lady stories are fictionalized accounts of situations Helena encountered or heard about during her time as a 'green lady' in Glasgow. Glasgow means, "that dear green place" and it was just that to Helena. In writing these stories, Helena was hopeful that her enthusiasm would inspire future midwives. She seems to have been successful, since both of her daughters studied nursing and one of them, who worked as a maternity nurse in BC for seven years, is now a midwife in North Wales.

Helena Joyce is survived by her husband Richard Barnes, two daughters, Morag and Sheila and two grandchildren, Rebecca and Jamie.

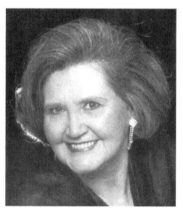

Helena Joyce (1939–2008)